Fabulous in a Fortnight

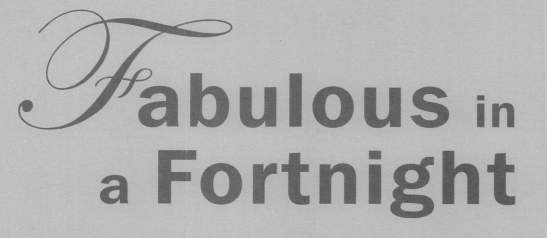

Fabulous in a Fortnight

The Day-by-Day Programme
– Shape Up and Lose Weight

MONICA GRENFELL

PAN BOOKS

To my husband Michael Grenfell

First published 1995 by Montgomery Books

Revised edition published 1997 by Pan Books

This revised and updated edition published 2005 by Pan Books
an imprint of Pan Macmillan Ltd
Pan Macmillan, 20 New Wharf Road, London N1 9RR
Basingstoke and Oxford
Associated companies throughout the world
www.panmacmillan.com

ISBN 0 330 43860 3

A CIP catalogue record for this book is available from the British Library.

Designed by Rafaela Romaya
Exercise photographs by Paul Bricknell
Food photography by Philip Watkins
All other photographs by Jim Marks
Printed and bound in Great Britain by Bath Press

Advice to the reader

Before following any medical or dietary advice contained in this book, it is recommended that you consult your doctor if you suffer from any health problems or special conditions or are in any doubts as to its suitability.

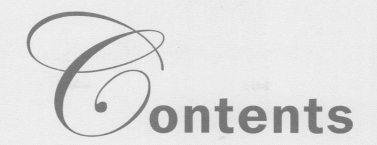

Contents

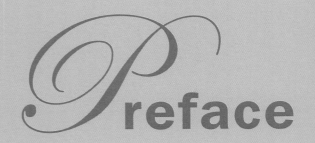

Preface

When I wrote the first edition of this book in 1995, it was a small, personally inspired manual on how to get ready for a special occasion. I had been going out with my then boyfriend for nine years when he suddenly said, 'Let's get married.' I decided to grab the moment and the man before he went off the boil. We got married two weeks later.

Granted, I didn't exactly look terrible before I started. But I was working hard and couldn't even get an afternoon off for a manicure. I decided to devise a proper plan of action so I wouldn't be spinning in all directions, but resigned myself to making the best of a bad job.

How wrong I was. I started a rigorous diet and stepped up the exercise. Losing half a stone wouldn't go amiss, I thought. You can imagine how great I felt when I emerged on my wedding day, looking and feeling completely sparkling, seven pounds lighter and with the clearest complexion I'd had for years.

I decided to write a book about my experience, but I felt something was missing. As a nutritionist, I have been at the birth of many wonderful weight-loss stories but despite impressive results, the dieters didn't always break box-office records for glamour; sometimes they were just smaller, lighter versions of their old selves. This was missing the point, and I decided to incorporate the 'it' factor into my book: how to help you lose weight, shape your figure and give you that certain something that makes people look twice. **Fabulous in a Fortnight** was born.

The book was a huge success. So why change a winner? Well, I became a magazine columnist, first for the **Sunday Mirror** and then, since 1998, with the **News of the World** I have ten million readers every week and thanks to the World Wide Web and email, I have contact with millions of people on a weekly basis. My website gets 200,000 visitors every month, so I am able to test out diets much more easily and I can get results from all over the world in a matter of minutes. People write in their thousands asking for more information about nutrition and diets and of course, the world of slimming has changed. Women have changed. The new **Fabulous in a Fortnight** addresses these needs and I have come up with a fantastic plan which I have been doing for years to help you lose half a stone quickly, carry on to lose as much weight as you need to and to keep it off for the rest of your life.

The integrity of the **Fabulous in a Fortnight** message remains dear to my heart: that beauty and image mean the entire effect you project, not bits of it.

A good body is the basis of fashion. A graceful figure is not only fashionable, but invariably healthier. Looking beautiful is as much about grace and poise as losing weight. And anybody who knows my writing will know that I don't just come up with pseudo-scientific results and a lot of baffling charts and diagrams to explain why you should follow one of my diets. Sometimes something works and people like it. My diets are tested thoroughly, not just for their effectiveness in weight loss, but to be sure they are convenient, family friendly and generally easy to get on with. As you will see, my volunteer testers are thrilled with the results.

The diet is called Food Separation. It works brilliantly and my diet testers have been delighted with the freedom from strict rules, adding up points, calories or grams and, of course, those tedious extra pounds.

So enjoy this book, let me know how you are doing and enjoy your new look. In just a fortnight, you're going to look fabulous.

*I*ntroduction

*H*ow is it possible to look fabulous in a fortnight?

If you're two stone overweight, tied to the house or are wracked with deadlines, a house move and a sick cat, it'll take more like a miracle in a month to get you anywhere near fabulous.

Right?

Wrong. Absolutely anybody can look fabulous. You don't have to settle for second best. It doesn't take a healthy bank balance or bags of free time. Most of us know someone who has all these advantages, yet still manages to look a mess. Everybody has what it takes to look good because that something comes from within. All you need to do is to recognize your good points, sharpen up your image, get a great shape and let your new-found confidence do the rest.

*W*e've all been there. It doesn't matter if you're wearing the entire Paris spring collection and have got the latest Louis Vuitton bag. It doesn't matter that you paid a fortune for your hair. If you woke up feeling fat, can't hold your stomach in and have a double chin, who cares what you are wearing?

On the other hand, we all know someone who can pull on a pair of jeans, tuck in an old shirt and look a million dollars. It's got nothing to do with spending a mint or having your boobs done. It's about style, and no amount of money can buy it.

Looking fabulous is all about feeling fabulous, and that means feeling confident. And it's hard to feel confident when you hide your midriff bulge day after day. I have known women fly into rages or refuse invitations on account of their stomachs. Everybody papers over the cracks from time to time, but you can't live like that for ever. You're living for now, not in the future. Don't spend your life saying you'll do something about your weight when this busy period's over, or when the New Year comes. Don't keep telling yourself you'll sort your skin out as soon as your college course finishes or your divorce comes through. In the meantime, you feel bad and your meter's running. Do something about it today.

Of course, you might argue that there is never a convenient time, your week is rarely 'normal' and it is impossible to get into a routine. I can predict that when a client hands me her food diary after two weeks, during which she has been asked to record everything that passed her lips, she will explain that those particular two weeks were out of the ordinary. Nothing was normal, she will say. That is supposed to explain why she binged on drink one day and ate nothing but crisps the next.

If nothing was normal, then this was her fortnight. It is what she ate. If you wait for everything to quieten down, you may as well wait for ever. It is a weak excuse to blame your own poor planning on your weight. Start today. Make times to eat and make everyone else dance to your tune. I promise it won't hurt, and what's the worst thing that can happen? You get slimmer?

You'll Never Be Caught Out

The fabulous woman never gets caught out. Even on a wet Saturday afternoon in the supermarket, taking the dog for a walk or putting out the rubbish, she looks great. My fabulous friend with the healthy skin and trim figure was once called out of bed in the middle of the night because her apartment building was on fire. Wearing an old T-shirt, no make-up, a roller in her hair and a slick of greasy night cream, she waited on the balcony for an hour while the emergency was quelled. Next morning one of the firefighters knocked on her door and asked her out. 'I think you're stunning,' he said.

It is completely worth it to look your best all the time. This is not as hard as it sounds. It is not about finding a new 'you' or putting on an act. It is about finding the best version of yourself. Going on endless diets, trying year after year to lose those pounds you've lost fifty times already, only to gain them again . . . you'll never have the struggle of dieting if you don't gain the weight in the first place. There won't be any mad, all-out gym sessions to get your thighs halfway decent if you just spend twenty minutes a day keeping them up to scratch. It is like keeping your home or garden in reasonable order. It's a mess when you buy the place and the garden needs six months to get it straight, but you never have to do that hard work again. Once your body is up and running properly it only takes half an hour a day to maintain it. Doesn't that sound like a dream come true?

High Maintenance Is Out

We've all heard about high-maintenance women. Frankly, if it costs so much and takes so long to look great, you're doing something wrong. And are the results really worth it? I've known scores of these women; they go crazy for the latest bag, belt or jacket, put themselves in debt up to their eyebrows and still look like nothing. You can't imagine why they bother. To be brutally honest, I have spent a few pounds myself on such nonsense but, fortunately, learnt my lesson a long time ago. Spending your way into being noticed does not work. You might be noticed, but then what?

I am going to prove that with a bit of organization and commitment, you can look fabulous in just a fortnight without having to book into a spa, spend thousands of pounds or splash out on a whole new wardrobe.

Yes, it's a bore not to drink. It's a bore to go to bed early with half a pound of cream on your face, but it's not permanent. It's far more boring to be fat and flabby and to know you'll wake up tomorrow, and the next day, looking and feeling just as bad.

True Beauty Can't Be Taken Off

Clothes count, of course they do. If you've worked hard on your figure, face and hair, the crowning glory is to put on something lovely and know you look terrific. Wearing something patently unflattering, over the top or unsuitable can undo all your good work. It is no good working for a marvellous figure then hiding it in a shapeless dress in a fabric that doesn't work. You can go the other way and wear clothes so amazing that everybody notices the outfit and not you. How many times have we had somebody say, 'I love your coat!' – or whatever. It is a great compliment and we should grab whatever compliments we can and be grateful. But having an outfit admired says nothing about you. Many people make this sort of remark when it is the only thing they can say. It might really mean, 'I love your coat because, frankly, it's the only bit of you I can find to say anything good about.'

Work for your total look. If every aspect of your outfit can be described in detail but no one can remember the colour of your eyes, this book is for you.

So we have arrived at the core of *Fabulous in a Fortnight*: making the most of your foundations; getting rid of those ghastly pounds and toning up. It's obvious. In this book we will deal with the following:

1 Your Body	2 Your Image	3 Final Touches
nourishment	posture	helpful tips
exercise	attitude	
flexibility	manners	
suppleness	charm	
tone		
gracefulness		

What Makes a Fabulous Woman?

I have canvassed hundreds of opinions to find out what people thought were elements of the fabulous woman. I asked all ages and both sexes. We all agreed that giving a fabulous impression means the whole effect, not just bits of it.

It means:

1 Being slim or curvaceous, with no bulges.

2 Having a defined waist.

3 Being well 'held together' with flattering clothes.

4 Having good legs and trim ankles.

5 Having a clear and healthy complexion.

6 Having glossy and healthy-looking hair that moves.

7 Having cared-for hands and feet.

8 Having good posture.

9 Having a good bustline, whatever its size. No drooping or spilling over a bra.

10 Having a bright and friendly smile.

The Bottom Line

One final thought. How often have you heard someone say that a girl was all right 'until she opened her mouth'? Or, 'She ruined it by the way she behaved at dinner'? Or some other scathing comment which suggests that beauty is more than skin deep?

This book is not an attempt to change your ways and personality totally, but we all have to acknowledge that sometimes it is our behaviour, or our speaking voice or general manner which can be off-putting. Long before I was a nutritionist, I trained as a teacher of Speech and Drama. I spent a few years teaching private pupils how to make the best of their speaking voice, which they felt held them back in some way in their careers. While this book will not address the drawbacks of a terrible voice or poor speech, we are usually the last to know, if we ever do know, that our voice puts people off. Do bear this in mind when you consider your final effect.

I have included a section on deportment because poor posture completely ruins a beautiful outfit and makes a good figure shapeless. There is a section on behavioural mistakes most of us make from time to time. Having said that, and if you consider me hopelessly old-fashioned, if your bubbly nature includes ripe language and extravagant behaviour and you feel it has never held you back in any way, by all means ignore my advice and press on. Be warned, however: if you are reading this book because you feel you somehow fall short in the popularity stakes, your relationships never work, and you never get asked to the right parties, you may discover this could be for some trifling reason you're not aware of.

Impeccable manners, a lovely speaking voice and beautiful posture never let anyone down.

You might also be surprised to know that most people feel unsure and nervous in unfamiliar social situations, even those who go to these things all the time. I know I can be. Good manners and charm never let anybody down, however, and knowing you look your best can at least remove that small anxiety.

If you knew it all, you wouldn't be reading this book. Even people who think they know it all are just as likely to find themselves feeling like fish out of water. Even if you aren't planning to go anywhere and are just using this book as a getting-to-grips-with-yourself improvement plan, the stories in the Infamous Disasters (page 107) section are a cautionary reminder of what can go wrong, despite our best efforts. The women I talked to were all experienced social-eventers who still managed to make some wild errors of judgement and ghastly mistakes, so do read these amusing tales of woe.

Of course, it would be a shame if we went through life so terrified of putting a foot wrong, saying something out of place or wearing the wrong outfit that we either never went out of the house or remained steadfastly rigid and po-faced at social events. Part of life's natural dynamics are the learning processes we go through when faced with an occasion which is outside our normal circle or experience. Different sorts of social events have their own rules, for example an artistic gathering and a sporting get-together. Etiquette exists to ease us through these minefields. People may mock it, but only by there being a common thread of manners and behaviour is it possible to slide effortlessly from one sort of situation to another without feeling embarrassed or out of place. The point of good manners and etiquette is to make others feel at ease. Don't ever get too hung up about an unfamiliar gathering. Someone is the host or in charge, and it is their responsibility to incorporate nervous guests and see to it that they are catered for. Just smile, which will encourage people to approach you, and look your best. You can do no more.

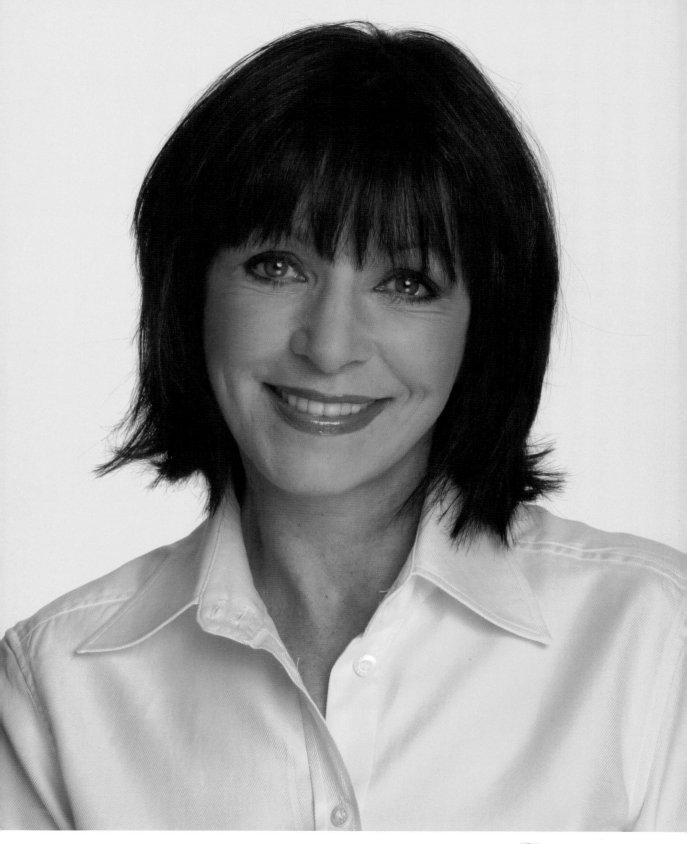

You've Got Just Two Weeks

People who have let themselves go always say that they haven't time to look after themselves. They are suspicious of people who manage to run a home, children and a full-time job and still look glamorous, and there's usually some bitchy comment about being able to afford it, having a mother-in-law to help, or a house-husband to take over. It's only jealousy. Everybody has twenty-four hours in a day, and compared to our mothers and grandmothers, who didn't have washing machines, microwaves or cars, we've got it made. No woman who considers herself efficient should have to admit that she can't find time for herself. Even in the midst of your many duties and responsibilities you can keep your looks, your health and your youthfulness. The trick is to organize yourself on labour-saving lines so you have more free time, not less. The secret is not to be haphazard. Designate a day for each task and discipline yourself to stick to it. This plan tells you what to eat, but in future make a weekly menu. It takes all the stress out of it. Haphazard shopping leads to impulse buys of things you then have to eat up just to get rid of them.

Maybe you live in the depths of the country and the nearest gym is miles away? Not everyone has state-of-the-art facilities up the road, and if you're managing on a windswept smallholding or have the builders in, a business to run and an elderly dependent relative, you won't thank me for suggesting you start the day with a ninety-minute yoga class.

However, good reasons soon become excuses. I was a young mother once, frequently managing on my own in a freezing cottage, miles from anywhere. In those circumstances, it's easy to feel there's no reason to look good, but you must soldier on. Children grow up, situations improve. In my day, exercise was a daily trot to the post office pushing a pram. Maybe ten minutes of stomach exercises. Being slim kept my spirits up because I reasoned that life might not always be like this. It might get better and I wanted to be ready when the call came or my luck changed. However drab or routine your life might be right now, getting and keeping yourself up to speed, toned, trim and attractive is like an insurance policy for the future. It might take a month to see a difference in your weight and toning can seem to take for ever to lose that vital inch, but there are so many things you can be doing in the meantime that really make a difference.

A new make-up trick takes minutes. A different hairstyle takes a matter of hours. Even a brilliant smile comes for free. Never underestimate the value of tiny changes and small efforts that can make a world of difference. Then, instead of flying into a panic when an interview suddenly pops up, or like me, you are suddenly proposed to, you will merely get your hair done, climb into a fantastic outfit and you'll be ready. Looking fabulous.

What 'Fabulous' Means to Me

I've already said that the basic elements of the fabulous woman are good legs, figure, complexion, posture, hair and nails. Add to this a friendly smile and you have a base which nobody can take away. But what do other people think looks fabulous? I asked a group of men for their opinions and here are the responses of a handful of them. See if you can find a common thread.

Andrew Dallas, 29, engineer
This is probably politically incorrect, but I don't like women to look like boys. Tomboys and assertive women turn me right off. So do bulging stomachs – how do women allow themselves to look like that? I don't have a problem with a few extra pounds, but hold them in, please!

Ken Fraithorne, 52, safety manager
I mourn the passing of skirts and dresses. Fabulous to me means a nice skirt and heels. I know it sounds like some kind of pervert these days, but it is just so rare to see real femininity. It doesn't mean a woman has to be meek and submissive – in fact it's incredibly sexy when a girl dresses fabulously yet commands the attention of a roomful of her staff.

Andrew Parker, 44,
newspaper and glamour photographer
I don't want to sound pretentious, but it's what we used to call at college 'aesthetic continuation'. That means a woman has many qualities which, put together, make her glamorous, but they don't all rely on each other. She can have bad hair, an off-day with her face or put on a few pounds, but the essence of her beauty doesn't suffer in any way. If someone is only gorgeous because of particularly stunning hair, or her figure, she's nowhere to go if they fail her, such as if she cuts her hair short or wears trousers.

   A woman should be able to make a lot of changes to herself and still look good, but I admit that it's rare to find someone with these qualities. My personal hate? Oh, believe it or not, I notice elbows and have a particular dislike for rough ones, or dry, 'goose fleshy' skin on the back of arms and shoulders. In my job I see it all, and you'd be amazed how many models forget the hidden bits.

Chris, 19, student
My mother is the most fabulous looking woman I know. She wears jeans and T-shirts and doesn't have much fashion awareness, but she eats incredibly well and has the most beautiful hair I have ever seen. She wraps it in hot oil once a week, and says she hates eggs but eats them because they're good for hair. I like her dedication.

Jeff, 26, catering manager
A woman's fabulous to me if she smells nice. I don't care about anything else. Nice meaning clean, not covered in perfume to mask odours. That includes nice breath and this comes from diet. I wish people didn't eat all that protein or garlic. Fresh breath, clean skin and nice-smelling hair – that's fabulous to me.

The Principles of the Grenfell Programme – How You Will Succeed

You are probably keen to get down to your diet. But first let's talk a bit about motivation. These are the principles of the fabulous in a fortnight programme

1 Decide on Success

Some women think of their figures as beauty injustices: they spend their lives punishing themselves with diets. Some women consider their figures walking laboratories for diet experiments. But the basic problem is that they decide they can't be successful. They say they will 'give a diet a try', rather than changing what they actually do about their relationship with themselves. For this is what it's about. Not their relationship with food, but why they keep eating it. You will succeed on this programme because every bit of you is being improved. So your starting point is not 'This is going to be so hard' but 'At last! I am going to be a new person!'

Ask yourself where you are right now. Maybe you are overweight, unhappy and totally fed up with your looks. You might be only a little out of shape, but desperately yearning for the person you used to be, with the shape you used to have. So ask yourself 'Where do you really want to be?'

Most people focus on the downside of taking control of their lives. They say, 'What if this happens and what if that happens?' People often get caught up in worry about being hungry. Instead of accepting this might happen, they take every possible precaution to have enough food to hand instead of thinking that food has been their problem all along. Then they move towards those negative thoughts nothing happens and they stay fed up and static.

If you make something positive your goal, like losing weight or getting firmer thighs, you will move towards that and each day you'll be a tiny bit further forward. Compare it to your hair growing – you don't notice it changing every day, but after a week, you can see a difference in length.

Change happens in a second: you say 'I quit' or 'I do'. It's happened. Change isn't hard, but you have to take that step.

Then how about the fact that people often dread a diet and assume it will be unpleasant? It is not unpleasant but you might start to focus on that. How many other, everyday things are not so pleasant but we do them? Going out in the rain? Getting up night after night to a crying baby? What about standing in line at the supermarket or waiting for a bus? They aren't pleasant. But we don't complain every time these things happen.

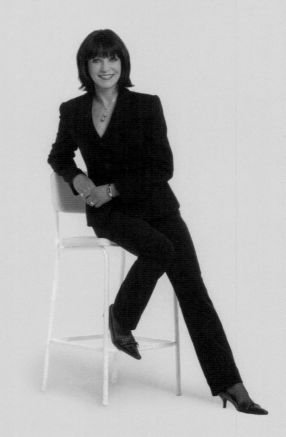

2 Respect Your Body

I once sat with a client for two hours and explained how her body worked. She expected a diet. I left her with nothing. She went away and came back two weeks later. She'd lost six pounds (2.7kg).

This was achieved with no more than her mental strength gained from a few basic facts. For the first time, she understood what food was for. Understanding and respecting your body's processes is the cornerstone of weight control. People don't often ask themselves why we eat.

All the time, day and night, whether you are working, sleeping, talking, eating or watching television, your body is working hard – breathing, pumping blood, repairing muscles. Did you know that new blood is constantly being made? New skin is formed and your nails and hair grow. How does it do all this? With the nutrients from the food you put into your mouth. So what's in a packet of crisps or a custard cream biscuit to make your hair glossy?

Next time you think of a meal, don't think of counting calories or fat or carbs. It is nonsense and avoids the basic premise that all proper food is good for you. Make a meal according to what it can do for you. Some diets give you a list of 'treats', they give you a food allocation allow for extra food if you exercise or have systems for saving food for another day. You are constantly bargaining and rewarding yourself with the very thing that got you into the mess in the first place. Rewarding yourself with chocolate is not a treat for your body. Putting that fatty, sugary little ball into your stomach is a nightmare for your body. A treat for your body would be an apple, a few grapes or a piece of fish.

Respect your body by never again allowing any rubbish inside it. Never eat meals that come from some factory. You get out what you put in, and the rewards are a fat-free, lean, energetic and healthy shape.

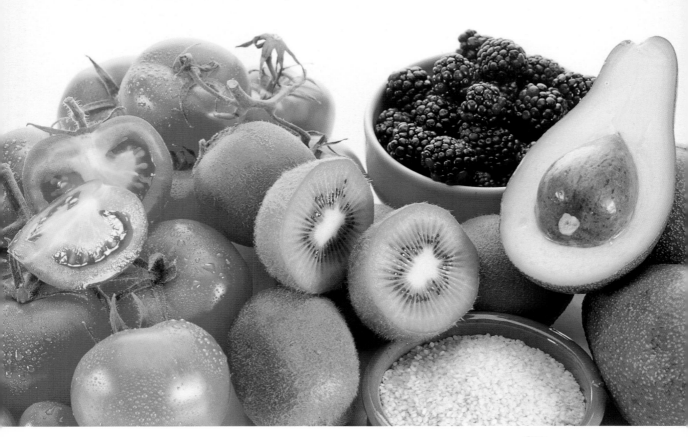

3 Eat for Beauty

Your top priority is to eat for your looks. Losing weight, getting a body to die for and toned, supple limbs are worthless if you look washed-out, have bad breath and are permanently exhausted. This diet is packed with nutrients that support skin growth, healthy thick hair and strong nails. Your internal organs need to be in good shape and your digestive processes clean and working properly – which keeps your stomach nice and flat and keeps cellulite well away.

4 Do Your Daily Dozen

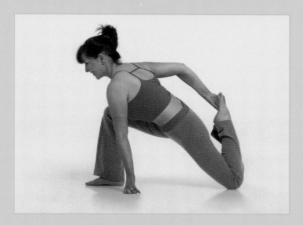

The twelve daily exercises I suggest will flex, tone and beautify your body efficiently and effectively. My daily dozen will transform your shape and give you suppleness, poise and elegance. They will help improve posture, lift your bustline, flatten your tummy and trim inches from all over. I guarantee you will love your exercises. Say goodbye to freezing cold early morning jogging and gym sessions. With the daily dozen, you will be toned and trim before most people have opened their eyes!

5 Observe Food Separation

Food separation is a trick of the trade that works. A few years ago I would have said this was nonsense. I dislike regimes that get too involved, which have people contemplating every morsel of food, worrying about what goes with what and whether something is organic. This type of self-indulgence is counter-productive and unnecessary, but food separation is different. You are eating entirely normal meals without any guesswork involved, but you separate starch meals from protein meals. It is not remotely fiddly, and my volunteer testers reported an average of two days to get used to it. After that, they were up and running without any guidance from me and I was thrilled to hear not just that they liked it, but that it helped them manage their appetites particularly well.

You can read how about the diet on page 22. The system works with your natural rhythms. You won't get obsessed with food, but by having limitations you will lose that tension most people feel when they are privately fed up with themselves and fed up with their lack of control. Food separation makes the decisions for you. I have given you plenty of meal ideas in this book and the fourteen-day diet spells it out if you need a firm hand to get you going. But once off the leash, you will go 'free range' without any trouble.

You should lose half a stone (3.15 kg) in the next fortnight. If you have a lot of weight to lose, you might lose more. But I do not want you to get caught up in the weight question. Yes, weigh yourself. It is an important part of this programme. But do not let the result affect you too much. As long as the trend is downwards it will continue to go down. Trust the programme and trust me.

Long- and Short-Term Goals

To be a successful beauty, you should behave like a beauty. Your first short-term goal is to do those small things that make you feel better about yourself but take little effort. Give your body the care and attention it deserves. Don't forget about it for weeks and months and then be surprised when your stomach is huge and your thighs are wobbly. It really isn't so difficult to maintain yourself, and once you've got to grips with your body it really takes very little time and effort to keep yourself slim, toned and supple. For the next two weeks your regime will be precise, so you get used to it and do not have to think too much about what goes with what and when. I do all that for you. Having to think about choices would be mind-boggling and stressful. So I have laid out your meals with a couple of options and hope this will ease you into it naturally. The long-term goal is for you to plan your own diet. Later in this book I'll give you more ideas to fit into most schedules. You can adjust this programme to suit yourself, so it fits into the rest of your life.

People fail on diets because their aspirations are short-term: we want to fit into a wedding dress; we want to look good for a party or a holiday. Then we slip back to our old ways. Once the compelling reason goes, there is no other reason. So how about the reason that you want to look fabulous all the time?

I too have felt defeated, depressed and dreary about myself. Staying at home can mean you think there is no reason to look good. Papering over the cracks became a part of my life; I'd discovered the art of dressing to hide flaws. So what changed? Funnily enough, it was talking to an elderly relative who was forty years older than me. 'So how are you going to spend the next forty years?' she asked. 'How do you plan to fill the time?'

How indeed? How much longer was I going to put off achieving my goals? Was I really going to spend half the time feeling dissatisfied with my hair and figure and the other half promising myself I'd do something at some indeterminate time? The children had grown up; I'd got married again and settled. So what motivation was there and, more importantly, with only one chance of a life, was this how I was going to spend it?

Life is not only too short; it is possibly too long too. Can you bear the thought of all this guilt over a piece of Christmas cake or hiding your stomach under a long jacket for another twenty years? If a diet hasn't worked for you, find another one. Have you really worked hard for that flat stomach or smaller thighs? For years I complained about my thin calves. 'No matter what I do,' I'd say, 'I can't get any shape into them.' Then I thought, But what do I do? I exercise every day for a week; they hurt, so I don't exercise again for three months. I haven't tried at all, and I have clients like that. 'I've tried everything for a flat stomach,' said one recently, 'and nothing works.' But she hadn't tried everything. She'd tried everything for a short time and then given up.

I can promise you that if you make something your long-term goal, set reasonable targets and stick with a plan you can fit into your life, you'll succeed. Changes you can make are:

1 Stop smoking.
2 Only drink alcohol on a Saturday.
3 Say 'I don't drink' – you'll start to believe it.
4 Stop eating one type of food – such as ice cream – and never have it again.

You can make your own list, but the key is not to fit things in. You don't 'fit in' taking your children to school or going to work. Find the time. Make the time! In just two weeks it's easy to turn yourself around if you have the will. Make your family understand that you wish to discipline yourself for a while, and try not to be too tense about it or make it an issue. Try not to tell the whole office or college that you're on a diet.

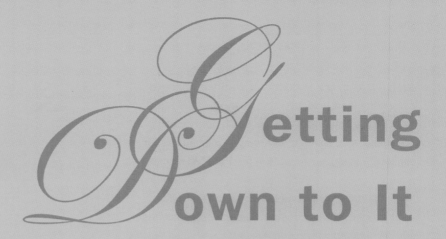

Getting Down to It

You must have been size ten once. You just went past it. You and everyone else on the planet are made exactly the same. We're all given a starter kit when we're born. How amazing it is that so many adults still have no idea what to eat! But not to worry. However much you have let yourself go, you can always turn back. However, this is not effortless, you can see where you are now and you know where you want to be.

Principles, Not Rules

Rules are fine for a short-term diet. But if you need something more effective long-term, rules will never work. Rules mean you stay the same person inside an exterior that wants to eat, so you will find get-out clauses. You will work out how to save food or make a meal with fewer calories, for example, so you can have a pudding. This leads to an obsession with what you are eating, constant awareness of calories and an unhealthy preoccupation with how you are feeling – hungry, full, satisfied.

Diet principles allow you more flexibility. If the principle is that you only eat food that will do something for you – nourish you – you know straight away that crisps are out; you know that avocados are fine. If you know you can only eat at mealtimes, there is no toss-up between whether to have a banana or some chocolate as a snack. A good principle is to eat the best things for your body, to nourish it and make it grow. Fruit is absolutely essential for fighting cancer-producing toxins and ageing, combating illness and viruses. Yet people still say, 'I don't like fruit or vegetables which is why diets are impossible for me.' Rules are about which food to eat; principles govern how and whether you eat, and that sometimes means forcing yourself to do what you know is best.

Sticking to principles means you are free to negotiate with yourself at a wedding buffet or Sunday lunch. Rules mean you will look at the roast potatoes and not dare to eat them. Rules are not healthy for your body or your mind!

You Eat Too Much For You

Obvious, but true. There is no such thing as eating too much, as such. It is about eating too much for *you*. Each of us has our own metabolism and while this can be manipulated and altered, it is still based on your personal make-up. Your metabolism 'sets' the engine room of your body which determines how many calories you need to stay alive and fuel your activity. The equation is simple: eat more calories than you use and you will gain fat.

Working With Your Body Clock

The usual advice is to eat most during the day and least in the evening, so you can try to work off your calories. But this goes against the natural working of your body, and in *Fabulous in a Fortnight* you will be eating in the best routine for your body to grow, repair and maintain itself.

Instead of eating calories only to work them off, the better way to eat is to use your stores, empty them, then fill them up when you are resting, and digestion is less laborious. In other words to put back what the day has taken out. There is a subtle difference. Think of it in terms of a supermarket after closing time. The shelves are ransacked during the day, shelf-fillers work throughout the night to stock-up so the store looks inviting and stocked, ready for the next day's rampaging shoppers. Shelf-fillers work better when the shop is closed. They can get on with their job. Think of your body like this. You are relaxing and enjoying your evening, then you sleep and your stocks are filled, ready for the new day.
It's obvious.

Another heartening part of my fabulous in a fortnight programme is your evening meal. I call it Meal 3. If you are a tiny bit hungry during the day, isn't it wonderful to look forward to a nice substantial meal instead of a small salad and grilled fish? Nice though fish and salad are, if you have just hacked your way through the rush hour carrying three bags of shopping and the trains were all cancelled so you're an hour late, do you really fancy a carb curfew?

You Forget That You Ate

I once observed some obesity studies. Subjects who lost weight in the clinic complained that when they left, their weight loss stalled. They were asked to write down what they ate. They were then brought back to stay in the clinic and fed what they had written down as their diet. They lost weight!

The conclusion was that they wrote down what they remembered eating. This is not to say they were untruthful, but can you remember exactly how much money you spent last week? We can remember the major items: the bills, the groceries or the dry-cleaning. We can't always remember the odd newspaper or parking fee. Over a week, these can add up to a lot. This is what happens when you try to recall the food you ate – you remember the meals, but not the bits of cake, the chewy mint, the slurp of wine from somebody else's glass. These add up too.

This is why the Grenfell system insists that eating is not part of any other activity such as watching TV or talking – at least not until you have your weight in check. If you must sit down and eat with a knife and fork and not think about anything else, you won't overeat. If the principle is not to eat anything between meals, you cannot forget that you ate.

Your Questions Answered

How can a starchy evening meal help me to lose weight? I always lose weight fast when I cut out bread and potatoes – now you're telling me to eat them!
Bread and potatoes cannot possibly be fattening. We are told they have a high glycaemic index and raise blood sugars quickly. Well, if you are incredibly hungry that is exactly what you need to do. Your evening meal will help raise your blood sugars and keep them stable for the whole night, which is why people sleep well on this programme.

Bread has no more calories per ounce than, say, fruit or lean meat. Two slices of bread have about 180 calories: an average salmon fillet has 300 calories. A jacket potato has around 400 calories: a steak has 600 calories. Calorie for calorie, starchy carbohydrates probably have fewer calories than good-quality proteins. There is absolutely no reason for a starchy meal to make anybody fat.

I have been on a diet for three weeks, I have obeyed every rule and I have only lost one pound. How can this be when I have hardly eaten a thing?
Your body does not know what a week is. Humans split lives into blocks of time and give them names, but your body simply 'is'. Bodies respond to routine: day and night, sleeping and waking, eating and using energy. They respond to seasons: warmth or cold. Changes are subtle.

You do not eat a cream cake, look down and hey presto! you are suddenly fat. Days can go by, drinking and overeating. Your weight stays the same. But those calories are stacking up and soon an extra pound of fat has accumulated. It is hard to notice at first. But losing weight works on the same principle. It works exactly the same in reverse.

I agree that one pound of fat lost in three weeks seems little. But in obesity studies, some people who came to a clinic dehydrated actually gained weight in the first three weeks of their trial because they were eating fluid-rich fruit and vegetables when they had eaten none before. Fluids are heavy. Five pieces of fruit a day can weigh three pounds. I strongly suspect that you were slightly low in body fluids when you started your diet and while fat has been lost, water has been gained. This is the obvious explanation if you are watching food intake properly, and I wouldn't worry. Stay with the plan and the weight will drop off.

I have been on a glycaemic index diet. I enjoyed it, but found it fiddly and I was eating six times a day. I keep giving up and eating too much, promising myself I will eat less later to make up. Why is this happening?
Your mind is in the wrong place. When you expect a diet to do the work for you, failure will follow. The glycaemic index system is workable and good science. However, you need to be very disciplined indeed to manage appetite control when you are attending to the detail of a system like GI. At the outset, you are continually referring to charts and as you explained, eating several small meals a day. I don't think this is a good idea if your self-control is poor.

The glycaemic index is a system of classifying carbohydrates according to the rate at which the blood sugars are raised. The theory goes that if they are raised quickly, as they are when you eat sweet things, white bread, potatoes and many other carbohydrates, they will fall quickly. This leads to cravings for more and more sweet or high-starch foods to make one feel better again, and this, they say, is what makes people overeat.

However, the theory is slightly flawed because the presence of protein lowers the GI of a food, meaning add a piece of fish or meat and you have a lower GI meal. Without delving into the finer points of this system, it is enough to say that weight loss and appetite control are hard enough without a lot of extra fuss. If potatoes made people fat, I would be a barrel. Weight loss has more to it than that.

Little and often diets work well for athletic people or anyone with a very active job. Not 'active' as in walking between offices several times a day or chasing after the children; these things have an appearance of activity because they are mentally draining. Slim women do not have a different physical make-up, but wanting to be slim determines their choices and decisions about eating. Slim comes first, eating second. The overweight woman puts eating first. If you are truly determined that you must lose weight, you just wouldn't eat that cake. Would you?

Blood-sugar levels have had a misleading press. The theory is that they are kept stable with low GI food and not allowing oneself to get too hungry. I find that three balanced meals a day keep blood-sugar levels just as stable and of course, a starchy evening meal does what it is meant to do: sends you to sleep. If you have a problem with food, the last thing you should do is eat frequently.

Take food out of the spotlight. Only focus on it during the times you are cooking or eating. Bargaining with yourself about eating less later or missing a meal is a very unwise way to go. Eating three times a day, with the option of having fruit between two of your meals, is the only way I know to lose weight and stay slim.

I have heard a lot about the 'natural' way we are supposed to eat. Some say we are natural carnivores and others say we are vegetarians. Which is right?
In a sense, it doesn't matter. Man has evolved. I once consulted a gastroenterologist for a book I was writing, and he told me that early man would have walked around with a huge stomach because he was capable of eating half a pig in a day. We are more robust than we think. Bodies are certainly made to eat and digest large quantities of meat, but primitive man did this because he had no choice. He also died very young of a multitude of diseases we do not suffer from today. So there is no sensible parallel between early man and us and you should forget all talk of a Stone Age diet.

There is a custom from the past which I employ in all my food advice. For centuries, each type of food was served separately, just as we have soup, then fish, then meat and then dessert. In the eighteenth century they separated the meat from the vegetables. You cleared your plate of meat before having a plate of vegetables. It is only in the past hundred years or so that we have eaten several types of food together on one plate, and only in the past couple of decades that we have had so many ingredients in one item of food – a pizza, for example.

I am not suggesting you eat everything separately, but if you have the usual modern problems such as irritable bowel, bloating and excess body fat, look to the blindingly obvious reason – eating too many different ingredients in the space of one meal. Here is an example:

· ham, cheese and pickle sandwich – bread, wheat flour, soya flour, emulsifiers, texture improvers, ham, preservative, cheese, pickle with onions, spices, peppers, tomato

- BBQ flavour potato crisps – potato, vegetable oil, salt, vinegar, monosodium glutamate (flavour enhancer)

- Low-carb chocolate energy bar – cocoa, sweetener, cocoa butter, emulsifier, glycerin, gelatin hydrolysate, polydextrose, soy protein, non-hydrogenated vegetable fat, whey protein, sucralose, colour

There are twenty-eight different elements in that one snack lunch, and I didn't count a drink. Twenty eight! That is a meal you might eat at your desk or in a park or while driving. You might even put it on the passenger seat and keep digging in for another bite. It's not surprising that people complain of a gassy tummies or reflux acid indigestion.

I don't blame you. We have to buy what there is. It isn't your fault that manufacturers stuff a chocolate bar with such terrible ingredients. But the *Fabulous in a Fortnight* programme has none of this food. Contrast it with a typical Food separation lunch:

- cold chicken with mayonnaise, colourful mixed salad, vinaigrette dressing – chicken, carrot, sweetcorn, lettuce, watercress, olive oil and vinegar

- plain yoghurt with sliced almonds – yoghurt, almonds

Nine ingredients, none of them chemically sourced. All natural. All mono foods – food which is one thing, not processed, only mixed like the vinaigrette dressing. Nothing added and nothing taken away. This is the basis of an excellent diet and this is why you will have a rich, enjoyable diet with plenty of wonderful food during your next fortnight.

I have such a huge appetite. I am worried that this diet won't have enough food for me.

Learn to know the difference between appetite and hunger. If you have just had a nice restaurant meal and think you couldn't eat another thing and then the mints come round and you fancy one – that is appetite. If, on the other hand, you come home from work absolutely ravenous and feeling shaky, and you only find two slices of bread which you devour without butter or jam – that's hunger!

Train yourself to respond only to hunger – at the start of this programme you must train how you respond, too. Reacting to every pang and rumble by eating is like picking up a baby the moment it cries. Break this habit. Learn to recognize that hunger can be held off until it is the correct time to eat. If you persist, you will soon only be hungry just before meal times.

The Correct Way to Eat

In my book *5 Days to a Flatter Stomach* I turned conventional wisdom and advice on its head. For years, you have been told to eat well for breakfast and lunch and to eat less in the evening. Some diet experts even suggest you avoid eating anything at all after 6 p.m!

This ignores the way your body uses fuel. So, people say:

'If I have eaten a bit more than I should, I make sure I burn the calories off as soon as possible,' or 'I have less to eat in the evening because I will be sitting down then sleeping, not burning off the calories. Eating in the evening turns food to fat.' This is total nonsense. For a start, our bodies use 500 calories between going to sleep and waking. It is what you eat and how much you eat that determines how fat you will get.

People who genuinely love their food never eat a lot. Plenty of food-lovers form clubs and societies and regularly meet at different restaurants to savour new tastes. True wine-lovers don't drink to staggering drunkenness. They take pleasure in savouring the wine. These people love food and drink and don't have a problem with it.

The problem begins when food becomes an obsession, and it becomes an obsession out of a kind of hatred. Obsessive eaters rarely notice what they're eating. They'll eat very little in public, saving their binges for quiet times alone. They say diets don't work and this is because food isn't being eaten for its own sake. Rather like smokers who wonder what to do with that yawning gap after a meal, dieters don't know how to fill the time if they're not eating. 'I can't have a cup of coffee without a biscuit,' said one of my clients. 'I can't sit watching people eat a pudding and not have one myself,' said another. Why not? It's not the biscuit or pudding they're missing. Eating can become a habit, and we programme ourselves so that coffee means biscuit, television means chocolate and a drink, shopping at the supermarket means squash and a cake for the kids.

I'm not totally against this. We all love our little rituals and they make life more interesting. But if part of being overweight is that routine of coffee and cake or telly and chocolate, BREAK THE CYCLE!!

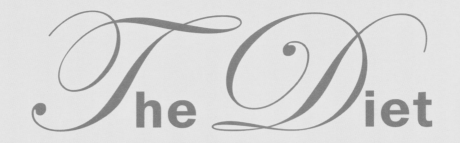

The Diet

The principles –

start as you mean to go on. From now on, you will be eating with beauty in mind. Beauty means getting rid of ugly fat on your thighs or that roll round your middle; it means a clear complexion and strong hair. Nothing on this programme has chemicals, additives or is processed. You will be amazed at the difference this will make to your looks in just two weeks, but over the following few months the effect will be dramatic.

You will have:
- clear, blemish-free skin
- stronger nails
- thicker, healthier hair
- clear eyes with no puffiness

You will also enjoy:
- twenty pounds (9 kilos) weight loss over less than three months
- a good night's sleep every night
- better moods, with no dramatic mood swings
- more regular, less painful periods
- an easing of menopause symptoms

You will also be eating what your body needs for energy, and that means eating in the correct rhythm. In the past you have probably eaten like this:

1 eaten a big meal or a naughty snack, and tried to 'burn off' the calories
2 eaten less after 6 p.m. because you are told that food turns to fat after this time
3 not eaten carbohydrates after 6 p.m.
4 kept nutritious snacks in your bag, in case you got hungry
5 worried that your blood-sugar levels would swing wildly if you went hungry

Well, if any of those old ideas haven't suited you (and let's face, it who wants to relax in the evening with nothing more than a salad?), you are going to be thrilled with me because I have good news. On this programme you will:
- eat after effort – that includes eating a substantial meal in the evening, when you are about to relax and then sleep
- eat a starchy, high carbohydrate meal after 6 p.m.
- have blood-sugar levels that will not swing because your meals will be large enough to sustain you for hours
- have as many potatoes or as much bread as you like

Food Separation – The Natural Way to Eat

Is this food combining? No, it's not. Those principles, which were made famous by Dr Hay in the last century, are sensible but intricate. They encourage an obsession with every mouthful and the system can be fiddly.

My diet is based on practical, simple and no-nonsense principles which are endorsed by everyday people like you and me. I believe we are made to eat all and anything, but a simple system of separating starchy foods from concentrated protein foods makes such common sense that I adopted it for my daily diet about two years ago. It is healthy, and as long as you observe the basic principles, I know you will lose weight and feel very healthy on this programme.

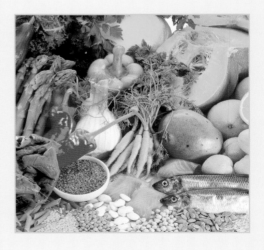

So What Am I Going to Eat?

Your body craves routine. It is on the go all day and all night, even though you aren't aware. Blood is being made, muscles are repaired, your digestive system is nearly always doing something – separating nutrients and sending them here and there to do their job. Your lungs work, your heart beats, hair is growing, cells are continuously dying and being made again. We are wonderful machines, yet we rarely stop to consider that all these processes need feeding. And not just with any old rubbish.

The energy from food is stored in the muscles and the liver. Gradually, you use this energy up. A sign that you need to eat is when you feel weak and tired. Having an empty stomach is a superficial sign and you should wait till you next meal before your eat.

It is highly unlikely therefore that food eaten in the evening will turn to fat, because the body needs replenishing and energy is still being used while you sleep. A hearty meal at this hour of the day provides nutrients for growth and repair. You rest and sleep, and during these hours your body can use that wonderful food to stock up again. Lots of lovely carbohydrates send you to a restful sleep.

The people who tested this diet, not to mention the millions of clients or readers who have asked my advice over the years, all reported such an improvement in their general health and well-being from something as simple as routine eating and starchy dinners that their friends, children, mothers and boyfriends were eagerly joining them. People who had not slept properly for years reported eight hours' unbroken sleep. Moody people told me they had calmed down and felt relaxed. Serial binge-eaters reported stable eating patterns and an end to their troubling habit. This is not just the ranting of an over-excited author by the way: getting a routine is the first step on the road to lifelong slimness and good health.

How Food Separation Works

Food separation keeps the starchy foods separate from proteins because proteins take longer to digest. A beef steak, for example, takes between four to eight hours to pass through the stomach. A potato or pasta takes one to two hours. Some foods are acid and others alkaline, and it can help your digestion to leave a period of time between eating these foods. By eating proteins for breakfast and lunch, you are avoiding blood-sugar slumps and you will feel more alert. In terms of bloating and better digestion, starchy food is pretty well known for causing a build-up of gas and while this is entirely natural, we tend to find it aesthetically unpleasant. Two small protein-rich meals during the day keep one alert and the starchy dinner fills energy stores at the end of a working day. It is plain commonsense and much kinder to your body.

The End of Endless Choice

Deciding what to eat can be a huge headache. I have tried and tested many methods of weight loss, including good old calorie counting, carb counting and low fat. Some worked better than others when it came to compliance. Being able to stay with a programme for life is the key to staying slim for life. Food separation scored top marks in my trials for compliance.

Food separation works because you don't have to think about calories or grams, just what goes with what. You are not denying yourself anything, just moving it to another meal. It is brilliant for controlling cravings because people don't mind the idea of having their favourite fancy at another time, rather than going without completely. By the time it is all right to eat it, the craving has usually gone. This method simply deals with your brain which, after all, is the most influential factor in a diet.

No Eating Between Meals

There had to be a catch, didn't there? You must never, ever, eat between meals or when you are not hungry. This is not as much of a catch as it sounds. Knowing you have a good meal to look forward to is an incentive to wait. When were you last really, truly hungry? Not just the 'starving' you might pronounce when your lunch is due but the truly cavernous, light-headed ravenous? I bet you haven't been ravenous for ages. I am ravenous every day at around 5 p.m. It doesn't kill you, because the energy is still there in your body from the last meal and your evening meal then tastes completely wonderful.

You might probably panic at the thought of not having snacks. After two days and several practice runs of getting through hunger pangs, you will feel calm and secure. It is quite normal to be panicky at the thought of not eating. But remember the bottom line in all this – you have two weeks to look great, lose half a stone (3.15 kg) and discover a better figure. It won't happen if you are not prepared to trust me.

Beat Your Body Chaos

Chaotic eating is the beginning of most dietary problems: irritable bowels, bad sleep, skin disturbances, irregular periods, weight gain and weight loss, yo-yo dieting. Most of the causes are eating quickly, eating at our desks, eating in the street, eating irregularly. The usual excuse is that people have no choice because their working patterns are 'all over the place'.

Well, my friend used to be like that. Then she was diagnosed with a serious illness and was ordered to take a certain medication at specific times of the day with food. This meant she had to eat at set times. Do you think she lost her very senior position or her overseas travel was in any way compromised by her new situation? Of course not. Forced to make decisions on her mealtimes, she did. Life continues quite happily and I can tell you, making a decision to eat at set times helps not only you, but others. Training other people to your timetable is a stress-reliever for all concerned. You will know where you are and other people will know where they are with you.

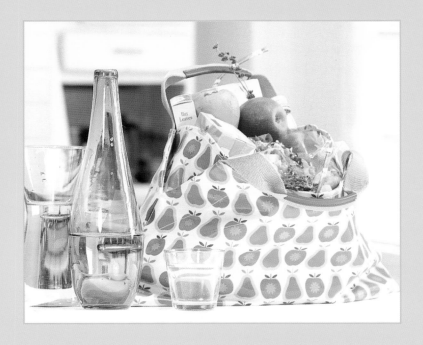

A Quick Guide to Your Diet

Your food is split into four categories:

- concentrated proteins
- concentrated starches
- versatile foods – go with anything
- fruit

PROTEINS

Proteins are split into two categories – animal and plant. They are necessary for the formation and maintenance of body tissues. There are three types of protein:

1 animal
2 lacto (dairy) protein
3 vegetable protein

There is always a major debate over how much protein our bodies need. Vegans argue that we can live on vegetable proteins alone. Vegetarians might insist we do not need the protein from meat, chicken or in some cases, fish. Traditional dietitians insist we need the high-protein content of animal proteins. One thing is certain: without protein we would fail to thrive.

Animal, lacto and vegetable proteins are digested in different ways. Animal protein comes from lean muscle and takes longer to digest than vegetable proteins like wheat or beans. For this reason, it is only the high-protein food items like meat, eggs and fish which you need to eat separately from your starches on this diet.

The usefulness of a protein to our bodies is determined by its essential amino acids, which are vital to us and which we cannot make ourselves. We have to eat them. The eight amino acids are:

- leucine
- phenylalanine
- valine
- threonine
- methionine
- tryptophan
- lysine

Proteins made from certain combinations of amino acids have particular functions which you will be particularly interested in, as they concern your looks. Collagen and keratin, for example, are directly responsible for giving your hair its strength and your nails their sheen. Other proteins affect your skin. Nutritionally, proteins are split into high- and low-quality. Don't think that low-quality proteins are not worth eating. They are. But ideally you should have the correct amount of high-quality protein daily and eat low-quality protein as an accompaniment to your diet, rather than as its backbone. High-quality proteins come from:

- meat
- poultry
- fish
- eggs
- soya beans

Low-quality proteins come from:

- nuts
- beans
- lentils and pulses
- rice
- bread
- pasta

How Are Foods Classed As High-Quality Protein?

A high-quality protein food must contain at least 10 per cent protein. All meat and fish have a lot of protein but bacon and some offal, for example, only have about 2–4 per cent protein. Don't get tied up in knots over this, as exact percentages will not make any difference to your weight loss, health or beauty.

Eating too much protein in the belief that it is somehow going to make you healthier is not only a waste of time; it can actually be harmful. Protein cannot be stored in the body so the excess is converted in the liver to glucose. A by-product of this is urea, which must be excreted and makes your urine acidic, which in turn leads to loss of calcium from the bones. In previous centuries, when a diet high in massive quantities of meat was commonplace, bone weakening was a symptom.

Despite the fad for high-protein diets and the huge quantities consumed by body builders who eat up to six egg whites a day and consume vast amount of meat in their attempts to build muscles, surplus protein is not stored as muscle. The nitrogen is removed and excreted, and the remainder is used for energy or stored as glycogen or fat. No harm comes from eating rather more protein occasionally, but don't make it a habit. You will gain weight in the long run from excess calories wherever those calories came from. I am afraid the fact that food is fat-free or healthy makes not a scrap of difference to your body when it comes to weight control. Excess calories get dumped as a waste product on your thighs, hips and stomach or a nice double chin.

How Much Protein Do You Need in One Day?

An average man needs around 50g/2oz of protein a day, the average woman needs about 45g/1.5oz. This can be derived from the following foods:
225g/8oz roast chicken
250g/9oz poached or grilled fish
25g/1oz nuts

Remember, too, that many other foods contain protein, such as pasta, milk, cheese and eggs, so it is hardly likely that anybody eating a Western diet would be protein deficient.

Vegetarians will find the programme quite straightforward. Breakfast and dinner are not a problem, but the high-protein lunch will have a little less choice, unless you eat cheese, eggs or fish. Tofu and Quorn without breadcrumbs are obvious choices, and these can be easily transformed into interesting meals with stir-frying techniques or salads that include nuts and seeds. In fact, using raw food principles (i.e. eat only raw food!) the most delicious and inventive crunchy nut salads with dried fruit, avocado and toasted pine nuts can be enjoyed by vegetarians every day. And by everybody else, come to that.

Omega-3 fatty acids are needed in small amounts, and can be found in the following:
a handful of walnuts
a 100g/4oz oily fish such as mackerel
2 teaspoonfuls vegetable oil

Omega-6 fatty acids, found in nuts, seeds and polyunsaturated oils, are needed in similar amounts.

STARCH

In the old days, carbohydrates were seen as stodgy and fattening. I have old magazines from forty years ago which expressly forbid fashionable women to eat starchy foods like bread and potatoes except for maybe one tiny portion a day. Starches are often thought second-rate. However, starch-rich foods are a main energy source and as long as you eat the right combination, during the hours that your body is re-stocking energy for the hours ahead, you will find starchy foods your best weight-loss resource. Hunger and energy dips are the usual downside of diets and the reason people fall off the wagon and binge uncontrollably on sweet foods. With a good starch-rich, complex-carbohydrate meal in the evening, you will break that hunger cycle.

The rate at which carbohydrates are digested keeps a sensible balance between blood-sugar levels for immediate energy and glycogen reserves for longer-term energy.

Where You Find Starchy Foods

Starch comes from vegetables. If in doubt, remember: if it is an animal, a fish or came from an animal, like milk or butter or yoghurt, it does not contain starch.

Foods HIGH IN STARCH
Above 80 per cent
- corn starch
- potato starch
- rice
- tapioca
- wheat starch

Above 70 per cent
- white rice
- brown rice
- wheat
- barley
- oats

- corn
- rye
- cornflakes
- spaghetti
- buckwheat

Above 60 per cent
- popcorn
- oatmeal
- bread
- noodles
- crispbread

VEGETABLES HIGH IN STARCH
- potatoes, especially fried and crisps
- horseradish
- ginger

VEGETABLES LOW IN STARCH
- pumpkin
- mushrooms
- asparagus
- green beans
- parsley
- peppers
- radishes
- parsnip
- chicory
- kohlrabi

VEGETABLES WITH NO STARCH
- all salad leaves
- fennel
- tomatoes
- turnips
- Brussels sprouts
- carrots
- cauliflower
- courgettes
- onions
- rhubarb

Where Fruit Fits In

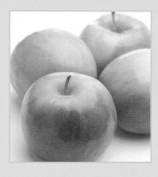

If you are going down the strict route of food combining, which we aren't, you would separate very acid fruits from the less acidic and combine them with either protein or starch meals. I can see why this is done, but again, it makes eating slightly obsessive and stressful. I am reminded that in other countries, people manage to live well and lose weight on diets that are completely different from our own, and presumably thrive on protein/starch combinations. The body is robust.

However, it's as well to be cautious. There are other reasons for not diving into any old diet and simply cutting calories. From my long experience of people's diet failures, they often gave up because they felt bad on the diet. Bloated, perhaps; edgy and irritable; not necessarily hungry. I put this at the door of populist diets that promise 'never be hungry again with our two-dozen daily treats!' which usually mean fun-size chocolate bars or bags of flavoured cheesy snacks at only 100 calories each.

Fruit is a dodgy area. You'd be happier if I said, 'Go ahead, snack on fruit any time you need a nibble', but I know how it makes some people feel. Eat plenty of fruit, definitely, but at the right times of day, on its own. It is well worth the effort of getting your head round the separation rules and, like a new job, it may seem hard at the beginning but you soon get into the swing of it and wonder why you ever found it hard. At this stage, people usually mention my book 5 *Days to a Flatter Stomach*. In it, I advise you to save fruit until the evening and not eat it during the day if you want to avoid bloating. This is a fact: the naturally occurring sweeteners in some fruits, especially sorbitol, not to mention the fibre and water content, is an aesthetic no-no for the elegant woman. So how come I am giving you a fruit breakfast on this programme?

Not everybody minds fruit. I don't have much of a problem with it, either. If you have eaten a lot of fruit all your life as I have, your body gets used to it and doesn't complain. At the start of a totally new programme, especially if you have had a truly dreadful diet before, your body won't know what has hit it. If your body is sensitive to the effects of fruit (and not everybody is) stick to yoghurt or milky drinks in the morning and have grapefruit and oranges for breakfast which tend to be kinder on your stomach.

Having said that, fruit is delicious, nutritious and sweet. Most people like fruit. So while there is this debate about the relative acidity of fruits, the most acidic ones are not those you would be likely to tuck into for pudding, namely rose-hips, lemons, sloes and cranberries. Blackcurrants are also a highly acidic fruit but as I said, it isn't a good idea to get too wound up over this. Starting with the barely acidic papaya, through mangoes and apricots to the fairly sharp grapefruit, all fruit is good. It is only a matter of eating it at the best time of day for good digestion.

I recommend that you keep fruit separate from other foods and eat it for breakfast and a couple of hours after your dinner. It makes a superb natural laxative. It is also something to look forward to when your idle thoughts might be turning to chocolate or biscuits.

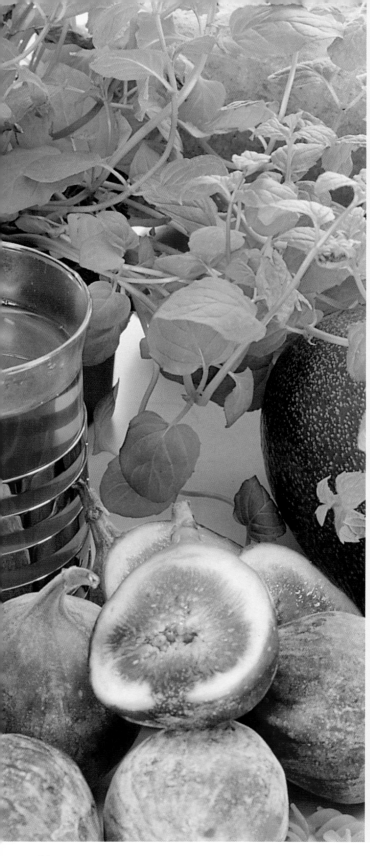

Top Foods On Your Beauty Diet

Skin
strawberries
carrots
nuts
milk and yoghurt
fish
tomatoes
peppers

Hair
eggs
cottage cheese
sardines
pumpkin seeds

Eyes
carrots
mangoes
apricots

Nails
Nails grow about half a millimetre
a week; a new nail takes about six
months to grow.

fish
cereal
spinach
eggs
seeds
wholemeal bread

Free Radicals and Anti-Oxidants

The body is made up of tissues and cells. These cells are made up of molecules. Within the molecules are electrons and electrons like to go around in pairs.

A free radical is a molecule with an unpaired electron. It therefore sets about trying to find another electron to pair with, and when it finds one, it leaves another electron without a partner, and so on. This continual search for a pair leads to a cascade of reactions, which in turn leads to cell damage and damage to the body. Free radicals start their journey of destruction because the body's cells are being attacked by poisons from food and the atmosphere. Indeed, two of our worst enemies are sunlight and tobacco smoke, which trigger free radicals and cause the skin ageing we associate with both smoking and sun damage, as well as related cancers.

However,the body is brilliantly designed to take on free-radical attack by the production of anti-oxidant defences – greatly primarily vitamins E and C. If you are at risk from radical attack – because you live in a polluted environment, you smoke or suffer from passive smoking or, God forbid, you sunbathe or go on sunbeds, your normal defences might not be enough. So, to prevent free-radical attack you should either take vitamin supplements, or, better still, eat a diet which includes plenty of foods rich in anti-oxidants.

Vitamins Which Guard Against Free Radicals:

Vitamin E
Vitamin E stimulates your immune response. Found in nuts, seeds, fish oils, seeds and wheatgerm. You do not need much of this vitamin – a handful of nuts a day or a tablespoonful of wheatgerm on cereal is quite enough.

Vitamin C
Found in all citrus fruits, cranberries, kiwi fruit, potatoes and vegetables such as peppers.

Selenium
The trace mineral selenium is a powerful protector against free radicals and cancer. Butter, Brazil nuts, avocados, lentils and shellfish are particularly rich in selenium.

Note

On this diet plan, you should not need supplements. The diet is worked out to provide you with everything you need for energy and glowing looks.

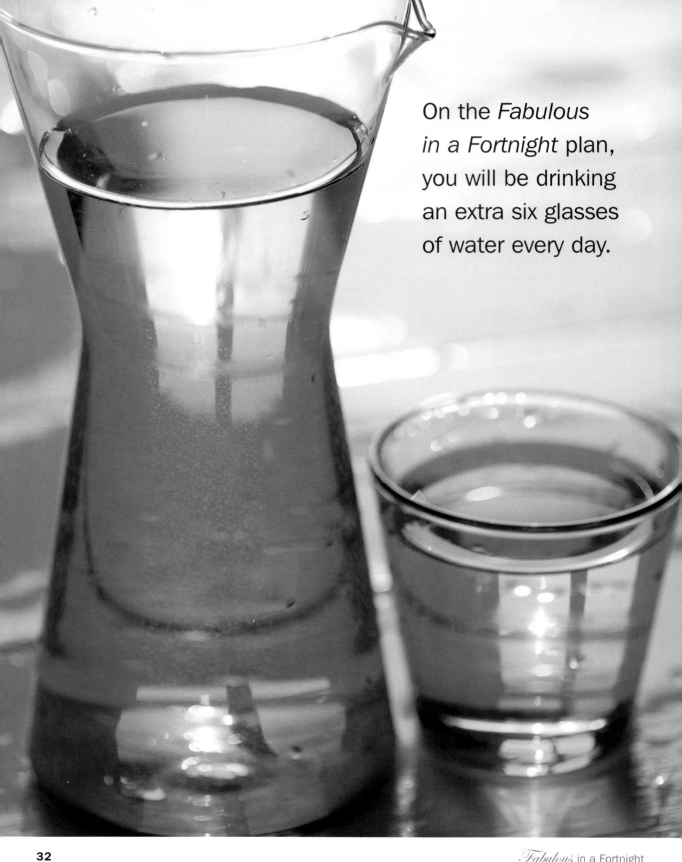

On the *Fabulous
in a Fortnight* plan,
you will be drinking
an extra six glasses
of water every day.

The Importance of Water

I cannot stress enough how important it is to take plenty of fluid.
'Yes, but I forget to drink!' one woman said to me recently. Or,
'I don't want to be going to the loo all the time,' said another.
Oh dear. I'm afraid that when it comes to drinking water – not the
most exciting drink – you have to view it like taking your medicine,
brushing your teeth or having your hair colour sorted out. Not the
most thrilling thing in the world, but we just have to get on with it.

Water is valuable to us in several ways:

1 It helps ease the passage of food through the gut, and is
   therefore vital to a flat stomach.
2 It helps flush poisons, which cause spotty skins, out of the
   system.
3 It helps 'plump up' your skin, avoiding a dried-prune appearance.

Your food also contains a lot of water, so if you regularly follow a
controlled diet and eat only one main meal a day, you will also be
lacking in fluid and should drink extra. Two signs of not drinking
enough are a blinding headache and lassitude.

Food Separation Tips

This really is simple. You have three categories of food: proteins, starches and versatile foods. All you need do is choose food like this:

- foods from group 1 and 2

- foods from group 2 and 3

- DO NOT MIX GROUPS 1 AND 3

- make sure your evening meal is from groups 2 and 3

Remember that you should only eat the fourth food category – fruit – for breakfast or a couple of hours after dinner.

Group 1	Group 2	Group 3	Group 4
PROTEIN	**VERSATILE**	**STARCH**	**FRUIT**
Beef	**Vegetables**	Bread	**Fresh fruit**
Lamb	**Nuts/Seeds**	Cereals	**Dried Fruits**
Pork	Almonds	Oats	
Fish and Shellfish	Cashews	Pasta	
Dairy:	Peanuts	Potatoes	
Cheese	Walnuts	Biscuits	
Cream	Brazils	Sweet Pastry	
Eggs	Pumpkin seeds	Gravy	
Milk	Sunflower	Savoury sauces	
Yogurt	Sesame	Sweet sauces	
Butter	**Fats and Oils**	Sweet pies	
Vegetable:	Butter	**Vegetables**	
Soya beans	Olive oil	Red, green, yellow	
Tofu	Sunflower oil	peppers	
	Low cholesterol spread	Radishes	
	Pumpkin seed oil	**Starchy Fruits**	
	Walnut oil	Bananas	
	All Pulses	Mangoes	
		Sweeteners	
		Syrup	
		Honey	
		Sugar	

A Few Meal Ideas:

You can combine foods from groups 1 and 2 and groups 2 and 3 but **never** groups 1 and 3.

GROUP 1: *PROTEIN*

WITH BEEF

Steak and salad

Stir-fried beef strips with mixed vegetables and soy sauce

Roast beef with juices (not gravy) and vegetables (no potatoes or Yorkshire pudding)

Cottage pie made with mince, onions, mushrooms, parsnip mash and fresh greens

Beef cooked in red wine with mushrooms, onions and bacon

Beefburgers made with onion, spices and egg

Beef stroganoff made with cream, mushrooms, onions

Chilli, no rice, served with grated raw vegetables

Beef curry and vegetables

Steak and kidney with mushrooms, onions and tomatoes

WITH FISH

The following served with green vegetables or salad:

Baked salmon with a pine nut and honey crust

Baked cod with pine nuts and honey

Plain oven-roasted halibut or cod with butter

Cod in white wine with mushrooms

Grilled fresh sardines

Baked smoked haddock in milk

Smoked salmon and avocado salad

Salmon and prawn pie baked in milk with mashed parsnip topping

Avocado with prawns

Salmon and corn chowder

Starch-free kedgeree

Crunchy seafood gratin

Poached cod or salmon parcel

Cod in lemon and caper sauce

Thai-style stir-fried vegetables with prawns

WITH OTHER MEAT

Lamb or pork chops

Lamb or pork curry

Lamb and mint burgers with onions

Roast lamb with mint sauce and vegetables

Roast pork with vegetables and apple sauce

Lamb or pork stir-fry

Lamb moussaka made with onions, tomatoes, aubergines and grated cheese

Shepherd's pie made with parsnip mash

Roast duck with orange sauce

Venison casserole in red wine

Roast pheasant or partridge

Bacon and walnut salad

WITH POULTRY

Roast chicken with vegetables

Cold chicken salad

Chicken and orange salad

Stir-fried strips of chicken with tarragon, crème fraiche and salad

Turkey burgers made with minced turkey and spices – nothing else needed

Chicken breasts cooked in white wine, mushrooms and onions

Chicken with pine nut and honey crust

Stir-fried chicken or turkey with pine nuts, broccoli and peppers

Warm spicy chicken salad

Coronation chicken

Spicy ginger chicken

Mexican chilli chicken

Country chicken casserole

WITH EGGS

Hard-boiled egg salad

Hard-boiled eggs with smoked haddock and spinach

Egg mayonnaise

Fine omelette salad

GROUP 2: *VERSATILE*

Cauliflower, broccoli and pepper salad

Grated carrot, white cabbage, sultanas and walnuts

Peas and sweetcorn

Lettuce, watercress and rocket

Waldorf salad

Cucumber and watercress salad

Strawberry and cucumber salad

Mixed salad with baby new potatoes, sweetcorn
 and peas

Fresh spinach and baby corn salad

Spicy vegetable salad

Spinach and avocado with yoghurt dressing

GROUP 3: *STARCH*

Jacket potato with baked beans and salad

Jacket potato with salad and mayonnaise

Vegetable pie topped with mashed potato

Vegetable stir-fry with sesame and pumpkin seeds,
 boiled or sautéed potatoes or 10 chips

Bombay potato salad

Wild rice and thyme salad

Lentil soup with French stick

Vegetable curry with rice

Vegetable chilli with rice

Pasta salad with avocado dressing

Spaghetti with tomato and vegetable sauce

Noodles with sesame oil, peas and broad beans and
 1tbs toasted pine nuts

Couscous with apricots, pine nuts and spices

Banana sandwich

Potatoes Anna

Pasta primavera made with stir-fried carrots,
 broccoli, peppers, and 1dsp crème fraiche

Bubble and squeak made with potato and cabbage
 with fried onion cakes

Veggie burgers

Falafel (chick pea burgers)

Potato cakes

Puddings, Desserts and Savouries

Puddings or desserts of any kind are forbidden on the fourteen-day programme. Eat fruit at least two hours after your evening meal, if convenient. However, if you are eating out or somebody has prepared a meal for you in their home, fruit is quite acceptable at the end of the meal.

To Drink

During this fortnight you may have

- unlimited water
- tea
- decaffeinated coffee
- cold water with orange or cucumber slices – slice a whole orange or cucumber and leave to steep. This is fantastic.
- fruit or herb teas
- one glass of wine per day (no spirits)

Portion Sizes

Portion sizes should take care of themselves.

You cannot have second helpings of anything on this programme, but I don't want to have you measuring and weighing anything. The whole idea is that you are calm and serene and not obsessed with the amount of food you are eating. Having said that, portions can make the difference of several hundred calories a day. Some portions manage themselves. An apple is an apple, half an avocado is half an avocado! It is harder when dishing out vegetable curry or calculating the size of a baguette. So I recommend these basic portion sizes:

- cereal 3 heaped tablespoons
- porridge oats – 3 tablespoons
- your plate – no bigger than 8.5 inches (20cm)
- Salads – a medium bowl. Try not to overdo the salads as a way of filling up – this is an overweight person's trait and needs watching!
- Dressings – 2 tablespoons vinaigrette, 1 desertspoon mayonnaise
- Casseroles, cottage pie, etc. – 3 tablespoons

Recording Your Progress

It is terribly important that you make a note now of your weight and measurements. So get out your tape measure and record your details for posterity.

How to Measure Yourself

Concentrate on the following points around your body:

Upper arms _____

Upper chest (armpits) _____

Bust _____

Under bust _____

Waist _____

Navel _____

Pubic bone _____

Hips _____

Upper thigh _____

Above knee _____

Calf _____

Ankle _____

Fill in this week's measurements, followed by next week's for comparison. Record your weight.

Note

You may find that in the second week your bust measurement appears smaller. This is more likely to mean that you have lost fat from your back rather than that your breasts themselves have got smaller! This is why I recommend you measure above and below your bust for comparison.

Putting It All Together

This is a good time to focus on the outcome. Somebody said to me the other day, before she even started her first day, 'I know this is going to get harder.' Why? We are only talking about food here. A few meals. An eighth of your entire day. Concentrate on how good you will feel, how slim and how 'together'. There is nothing that can possibly come out of the programme other than a more beautiful you.

So what if things don't go to plan? Well, for the first two weeks, you must be sure they do. Don't deviate from the system for two weeks. Stay away from anybody and anything that will derail you. Don't go out with people who are a bad influence. If you are getting ready for an important event, letting go with alcohol or fatty food is a crazy thing to do. You might as well not bother and look short of your ideal for ever. So stay with the programme, then you can add variations as and when you choose in the future.

Your meals should be:

Breakfast	Protein or fruit
Lunch	Protein
Dinner	Starch

You don't count calories on this diet, but calories always count. There is a big difference between the person who needs to lose half a stone (3.15 kg) and the person who wants to shed four stone (25 kg). If you have a lot of excess body fat, you have a lot of energy to spare. Therefore I have no problem with a very low calorie (VLC) diet. This will nourish you with good foods but force your body to dig into those fat stores and make them disappear!

The VLC options are marked * in the menu plans (see pages 86–98). There is a reduced calorie option for breakfast of just two oranges and a grapefruit. You can have this every day if you like, but as citrus fruit has no protein, I do suggest you vary this with eggs or fish at least twice a week.

Do not worry about eating VLC. Diets thirty and forty years ago always had far fewer calories than they do today and people did not have serious weight problems, either. I have dozens of friends who used to diet on 1,000 calories a day and they are all happily in their forties and older, still slim and gorgeous and not remotely aged or haggard or malnourished from their experiences. I have eaten a very low-calorie regime for years and my recent bone scan revealed the bones of a young woman – and I have never taken hormones. As long as you have a portion of milk, fruit, fish and a few nuts plus a good daily dose of high-starch food like potatoes, I know you will be healthier, happier and slim. So if you have more than a stone (6.3 kg) to lose and are not worried about getting too bored with your diet, I heartily recommend the VLC options.

Problems and Pitfalls

The following are not problems or pitfalls at all. But at the start of any new regime, there are a hundred questions: what if this and what if that. It's only natural. One of the first questions is, 'What if I want a protein meal for dinner?' Another is, 'What can I do when eating out?' and finally, 'If I want to lose a few pounds, I usually cut out bread and potatoes. Won't the starch meals make it impossible for me to lose weight?' So here are the answer to those and a few other questions.

What if I want a protein meal for dinner?
After the first two weeks, fine. Switch around the meals to suit yourself.

I don't understand the difference between carbohydrate and starch. Will any carbohydrates do for meals and must they all be kept separate from proteins?
All starches are carbohydrates but not all carbohydrates have starch in them. Look at the lists on pages 28 and you will see the highest-starch vegetables. These are the ones to keep separate from proteins, though fruit, a carbohydrate, also needs to be separate.

If I eat fruit with a crumble or pastry topping, does this still have to be kept separate from my main meal?
I'd hope you weren't eating fruit crumbles or pies anyway on your fabulous in a fortnight programme! But on the maintenance programme you can have one tablespoon of a fruit crumble or pie with crème fraiche after a starch main meal.

How often should I weigh myself?
Every week. You look at your face and hair every day, check your nails to see if they need filing, check your eyebrows don't need tidying or your legs aren't sprouting more hairs than you'd like. Why not check what your body weighs too?

I work shifts. How can I manage this programme when I come home at 6 a.m.?
It's easy. As long as you observe the principles. See how your body feels. I suggest a starch meal when you come home and before bed. A good bowl of porridge with milk will settle you to a good sleep. Have a protein meal on waking.

Can I have two protein meals a day on the maintenance programme?
Yes. But do remember that protein is not so efficient at providing energy and too much protein isn't a good idea for your body (see page 27). You only need very small amounts per day, so keep portions small.

Can I have two starch meals?
Absolutely, but the same rule applies. If you do this, have some yoghurt with your fruit or extra milk in a coffee as you will need the protein.

When I reach maintenance, can I eat fruit as a snack between meals?
Fruit is not disallowed and if you were to sit down and cut up an apple into eight slices I would say fine. But most people grab an apple and chomp through it in the car or at their desks and it is this that I find disconcerting. Snacks are not necessary for the well-nourished person. However, if you miss a meal and are stuck on the motorway in a tailback then of course – it's better to eat grapes than a packet of crisps.

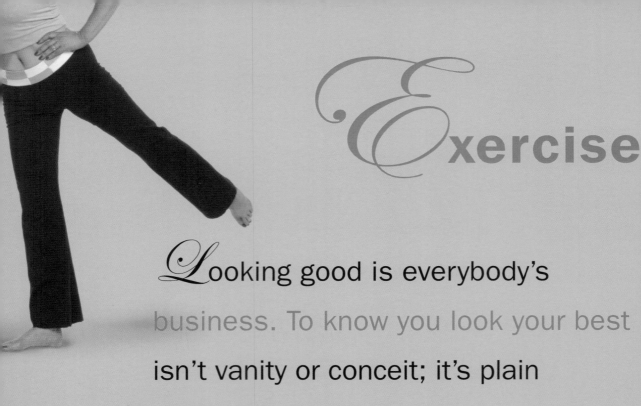

*E*xercise

*L*ooking good is everybody's business. To know you look your best isn't vanity or conceit; it's plain common sense. It gives you confidence and that helps others because you're simply nicer to be with. Exercise must be part of your day. Every day. If your usual exercise routine is a crash programme followed by weeks of nothing, ending up with a bad back, it's not surprising you don't have the body of your dreams.

However, if I am jumping to conclusions and you love exercise but don't look as fabulous as you'd like, no problem. We all have to work harder on particular areas. Hips are difficult because clothes solutions are hard to find. Waists are non-negotiable. However much we debate the comparative merits of big bottoms over small, and natural breasts versus big and silicone, a big waist is never in fashion. Time spent working for a good shape is never wasted.

We talk about our bodies when we mean our figures. Let's think about the 7/8 of your body that makes your figure. Here are some facts about it:

Your figure can be made slim

If I had a fiver for every time a woman said to me, 'I'll never be slim – I was made this way,' I'd be very rich. Everybody says it. It's not true, but try telling that to a mature person who has dieted for forty years. We can all make ourselves slim if we are determined enough. Losing body fat is one thing, but the real shaping comes from exercise. Finding a bulge is no longer there makes a huge difference to how you feel, even if the scales only register a so-so loss.

Exercise won't alter your weight to any noticeable degree, but it can change your figure taking inches off your arms, midriff and hips by toning and tightening the outer layers of muscles. Exercise has other benefits, too: stress release, outdoor interest, natural tranquillizing and beauty benefits; these are a few of the added benefits.

Your figure can be made to curve

A female body that doesn't curve doesn't really count as a figure. If you need to gain a bit of shape here and refine it down there (and which of us doesn't want that?), you need to do specific exercises in those areas. We all bear the inherited figure quirks that make us who we are and not clones of everybody else. I always loathed my narrow shoulders until my wise son pointed out that this is what Monica Grenfell's shoulders look like. Don't be put off when I tell you that the slow transformation took four years. You are changing your body's natural inclination but its only inclination is to a muscle type and build, not a fat gain. Fat gain is entirely voluntary.

I can assure you that in the longer term, if you absolutely want to have fuller calves, a perkier chest or thinner waist, you will.

Your figure can be made firm

Many women think they are overweight when they are simply untoned. The most important thing about muscle toning is that it can be done at any age – muscle is there anyway and it has no idea how old you are. It is never too late to improve muscle tone.

Your figure can simply look better in seconds

Slumping, slouching, head thrust forwards, shoulders hunched – these destroy a good figure. In fact, bad posture can spoil a lot of your fine work on your figure and is responsible for more figure faults than your figure should be blamed for. Good posture carries the body beautifully.

Your figure can learn to move well

Are you nervy? Do you wear poor shoes? Are you totally comfortable and at home in that outfit? Discomfort and self-consciousness freeze the body. Daily limbering and stretching will help unfreeze you.

Your figure can be allowed a few secrets

How many of us have been congratulated and complimented on our look and shape, when we know only too well that underneath lie a few shocking bulges or extra pounds. Delegate a bit of responsibility to your clothes. A good foundation and sense of style, a spirited walk and a firm shape will render a few pounds completely unimportant.

Getting Started

I assume you are not a total fitness novice. Given the day and age, most of us have flirted with exercise at some stage, but I am concerned that exercise has come to mean nothing more than fitness. In fact, most people I meet, who are perhaps overweight and out of shape, have no real idea what they are exercising for. 'How much exercise do you think I should try to fit in?' is the usual question. Or maybe, when I suggest adding exercise once a weight-loss regime has been established, 'Of course – what did you have in mind?'

It should be more a case of what they had in mind. They were hoping I'd hand them a sheet of exercises or a programme. Now, I am about to give you a programme, but that's because I haven't met you. Generally speaking, exercise isn't some sort of plan but a part of everyday routine. It should be woven into your life so you miss it when it is skipped. But much more important, and because this book is about your total look, I want to talk about exercise in the context of youthfulness and looking beautiful at any age.

The young look is fast becoming a lost look. Inactive people show signs of age much faster. We can't help getting old, but we can control ageing. Sometimes this is no more than a look of bounce and brightness; often it amounts to somebody's perky posture and lightning speed of walk. It can be a sense of purpose that transmits itself to others. Many very old people lose their purpose and it is sad when it shows. When you are young, however, it is doubly sad to look as if there is no reason to go anywhere and nothing to do when you arrive. It is unattractive.

Changing this so you appear confident and purposeful is as simple as limbering up, stretching and gaining control of your muscles. You do not have to be a keen runner or have defined biceps. Everyday exercise will sharpen you up, lift you mentally as well as physically. Eventually you will look as if you spend time training daily and people will be saying – 'Hey, you've been working out!'

Incidental Exercise

There are two types of exercise one of which, incidental exercise, is the kind you can't help doing: getting into the bath, bending to feed the cat or walking to the dustbin. It all counts. I want you to double the amount of incidental exercise you do. For example, some people hardly ever get off the sofa and get everyone else to do the fetching and carrying and making of coffees. Try carrying your bags of groceries instead of using a shopping trolley. Park in the furthest slot at the supermarket and run to the door. Nothing dramatic happens after a week of walking for your newspaper but, you know, these efforts mount up. They make you a better person. People stop whining for things to be brought to them and go upstairs for them themselves. Over a period of time, real shape benefits become apparent as thigh muscles tone and lengthen, backs lose bra-flab and your jeans feel loose on the thighs.

I often observe clients who are mystified about their lack of weight loss, and note that they take ages to do everything. They move like an elephant. While it is admirable to be unhurried and placid, it is often the root cause of weight problems. Everyday, incidental exercise should be done with this added energy, and you will find is it not only more pleasant and invigorating to be brisk, but it takes less time. You have more precious hours to devote to yourself, a beauty job perhaps, or your even better beauty aid, relaxation.

Another bonus from exercise is fresh air. Oxygen is a great beautifier. Look at the slabby, thick, pale skins of people who sit indoors and smoke (or inhale other people's smoke). I used to smoke so I am allowed a comment. I looked dreadful and it took a while to gain my complexion back. Exercise is a tranquillizer. How many of us fall into bed tired but not sleepy, to toss and turn for hours, waking feeling more stressed than before.

Specific Exercise

The other type is specific exercise which, combined with a strict diet, should give you a lean, trim and curvaceous figure. However, depending on the life you lead, it is unlikely to use all muscle groups to full advantage. Take walking: it uses your legs, hips and buttocks but not to any taxing degree and it certainly doesn't use your chest or abdomen. The leg muscles do not even get a thorough workout. Now, whether or not you need a thorough workout is another matter. In the days when we were clothed from top to toe and no more than an ankle was in view, toned muscles had very little relevance. We became interested in our bodies when the clothes came off. The more we show, the more we worry about what we show. There's no hiding place for a wobbly inner thigh in a bikini!

But let's assume that you want to look as good underneath as you do on top. Specific exercise targets areas you want to change, plus it uses the full range of your joints. This is important. Pain and strain are felt in unused parts of the body. Here are examples of movements I bet you hardly ever make, but which your joints are capable of:

Shoulder – the only joint that can do a complete circle. When did you last do this?

Knee – can hinge completely backwards so the foot touches the buttocks. Can you do this?

Hip – can move your leg out to the side at 90 degrees, forwards and backwards too. It can flex so far that your whole thigh can rest on your chest when lying down.

It is a good idea to put yourself through your paces at frequent intervals by trying these moves. Think of it as taking that old car out of the garage from time to time. Cars run better when they are exercised. So do you.

Aerobic exercise

Unfortunately, aerobics has fallen ever so slightly out of fashion. I do love those sociable classes and they are a fantastic way to get you out of yourself as well as improving your figure. These days I run to buy the newspaper – four miles there and back – or I cycle to town, a ten-mile round trip. You can't beat the idea of combining a task with exercise. I would still use a treadmill quite happily if the weather was dreadful, but if you can get out and walk briskly, rake leaves or something else to get the heart pumping and put a glow in your cheeks, all the better. It gets a job done too.

Running

When we grow up and give up our childish running, that's when our figures start the gradual process of ageing. Run for the train, run up the escalator. I didn't start running until four years ago. I won't tell you the age I was, but it was an age when most women say, 'I don't suppose there's any hope of being slim, not at my age.'

Despite my fitness, it was not something I excelled at. My first few goes were pathetic, I was embarrassingly breathless after a few metres and I couldn't see the point. Then I had one of those landmark birthdays. I decided to try again. This time I wore top-of-the-range running shoes and I ran more slowly. I had been going far too fast and with the wrong action. I started to run just 100 paces and walked 100. This became 200. One morning I realized I hadn't stopped for nearly a mile. I'd found my confidence.

Just so you don't think I am some kind of superwoman and I am planning the London marathon, that all took more than a year. Now I run every other morning. I wouldn't want to run more than four miles. It takes about forty minutes and is the best start to a day. Get a proper sports bra. Buy the best running shoes you can afford. They will make all the difference and soon, I know, you will be enjoying the start of every day, feeling positive and energized.

Stretching

Stretched limbs look leaner and a supple body is youthful. Stretching does marvellous things to the body that are almost an optical illusion. I know a woman of only 5ft 1in tall whose legs look the longest ever. She dances and stretches them daily. Stretching tones and gives you a command of your body. Stretched muscles are strong but lean, rather as a ballet dancer's shape is lean but not thin. It is a wonderful, chic and stylish look, and I have added some stretches to your Daily Dozen which will improve your figure dramatically during this fortnight.

Walking

Nobody was ever sorry they took a nice brisk walk. People are only sorry they didn't. Start by walking as fast as you can for fifteen minutes. Then walk briskly back. See how far you walked. You should be able to walk at least one and a half miles in half an hour, which is three miles an hour. With time, I would like you to work up to two miles in those thirty minutes. That's brisk!

Try also to alternate that with cycling. Walking only uses some muscles; others like your stomach, arm and back muscles are less active during walking. If you go to work, have a break at lunchtime and have a walk, whatever the weather. Sitting in the office will dull your mind and make you feel sleepy. Don't work through your lunch hour. What can be more important than feeding your poor body, which is crying for a bit of love and attention? You give it a packet of crisps and tell it to crack on for another four gruelling hours. We all get the bodies we deserve, so getting a bit wet or leaving that report for half an hour is well worth it if you end up with a figure you can be proud of. In any case, exercise helps concentration and you are better for that break, some fresh air and a boost to those snoozing joints and muscles and a mental break from endless words on a page.

Relaxation

Working your body week to week, day to day is counter-productive. Many women overdo the exercise and are terrified that if they stop, they will become fat and flabby.

Well, let me tell you something: over-exercising turns into self-obsession and shows a lack of confidence. Being fit and healthy are absolutes. You cannot be healthier than healthy or fitter than fit, and if you have a nice shape, you need very little effort to maintain it. Certainly exercising more and harder does nothing.

You need to realize that improvements and changes happen when exercise stops.

I like the analogy of a cake being baked. You mix and chop and add this and that and beat and stir – but the final result happens when you leave it alone, put it in the oven and wait to see what happens. The results come when you stop. I always advise my readers to eat well in the evening and allow the food to do its work while they are relaxing and sleeping. As long as the food is good and not some takeaway junk, the nutrients from that meal will replenish supplies, maintain muscles and feed your brain.

Brain tiredness results from your brain flashing endless messages to muscles. One muscle can do forty contractions a minute when you are exercising and that's a lot of signals from your overworked brain. Your brow gets wrinkled through worry, your lips puckered through concentration as you pound the treadmill. Stop and let go. Relaxation will do more for your look than exercise. Know when to rest.

The Daily Dozen

I love the daily dozen. It does all you need to be supple, strong and toned, without pumping you up. Old-fashioned exercising from the 1990s required a lot of body building and resistance work. It built muscle. Fortunately, a beautiful figure does not need defined muscles. It needs to be fat-free, with a defined look.

To this end, a beautiful body needs plenty of stretching, bending and toning. This programme should be done every day, in addition to general aerobic exercise, walking, cycling and so on.

What an Active Life Does for Your Beauty

Everybody knows that a good circulation helps skin and hair look fantastic. When the blood is pumping round, it gets to the ends of the capillaries and this makes you bloom. Do try to spend a little time every day getting your heart pounding and lots of lovely oxygen into your blood. It will make all the difference to your looks.

What if You Find it Hard to Exercise?

As I said at the outset, exercise is not as valuable as we would like it to be, when trying to lose weight. It cheers, it lifts depression and it helps shape muscles. If you are older or not physically capable take as much exercise as you can. In any case, the Daily Dozen has several modifications for people who cannot do the full programme.

TIPS

1 Do these exercises early in the morning before breakfast or in the evening, before you eat.

2 Warm up first.

3 Wear loose clothing.

4 Be warm, not too cold.

5 Breathe slowly and steadily.

1 Feet and Hands

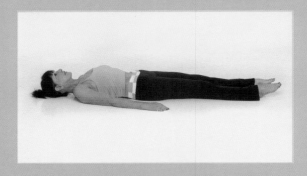

Let's start with the extremities: beautiful ankles and hands need exercising.

a While still in bed or lying flat on the floor, lie with your arms by your sides. Straighten your legs and lock your knees. Flex your feet.

b Point and flex the toes as hard as you can, staying in each position for a few seconds.

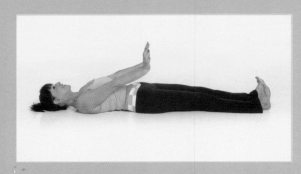

c Make the movement count. Really feel as if you could go further!

d Raise your arms right above your head and stretch. Arch your back. Bring your arms above your body and flex the wrists, as with the feet, in both directions. Try to make them go as far as they can.

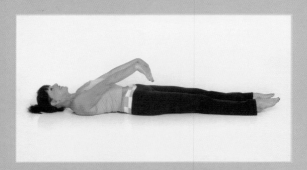

e Circle the wrists slowly ten times each way.

2 Wake-Up Stretches

Stand by an open window
and take three deep
breaths. Bend slowly to
each side to wake up your
torso.

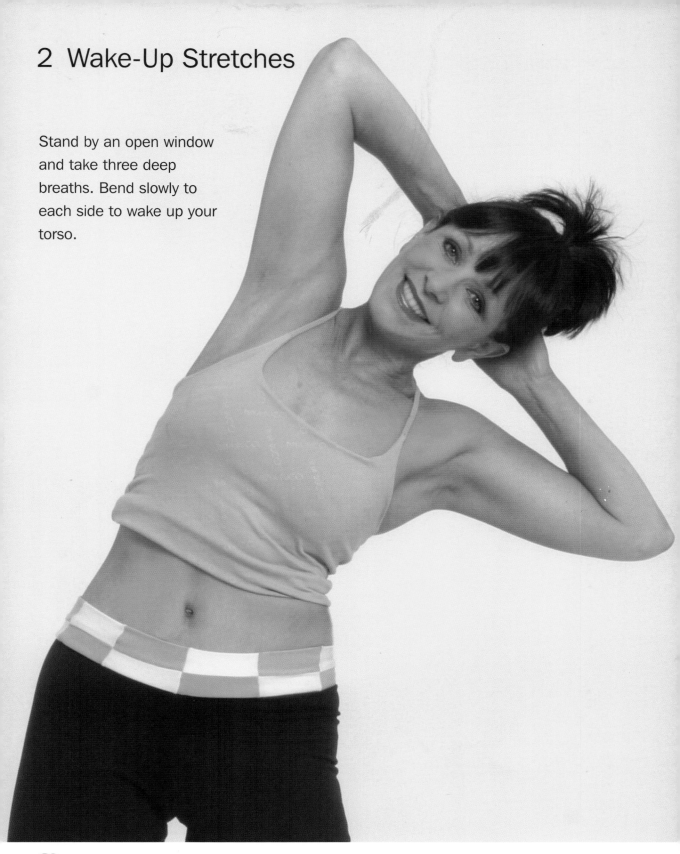

3 Shoulders

Circle your shoulders six
times forwards, and six
times backwards. Repeat,
circling your arms.

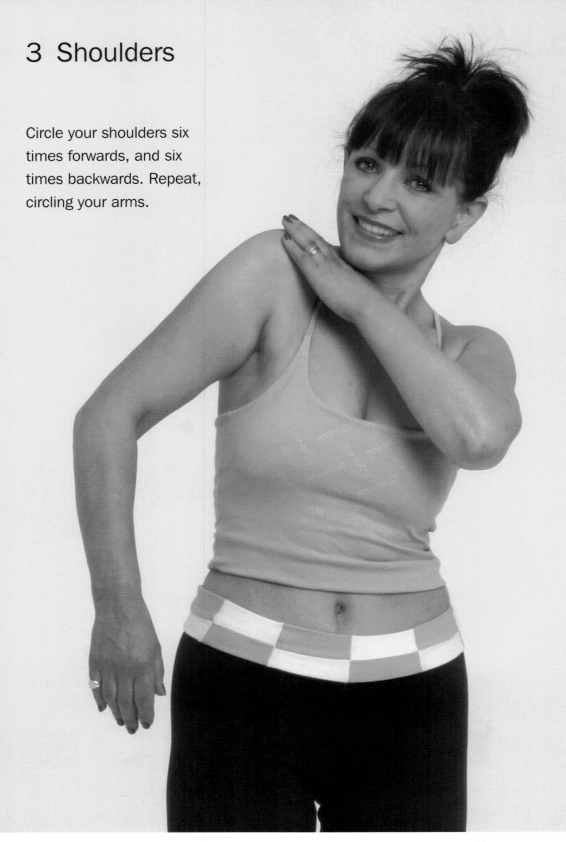

4 Hips and Legs

a Stand sideways to a chair and hold on to the back for support.

b With an easy swing allow one leg to swing back and forth ten times.

c Try to increase the movement each time, trying to go as far as possible.

d Keep your torso upright and rigid. Let your hip do the work.

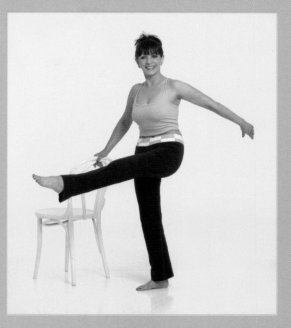

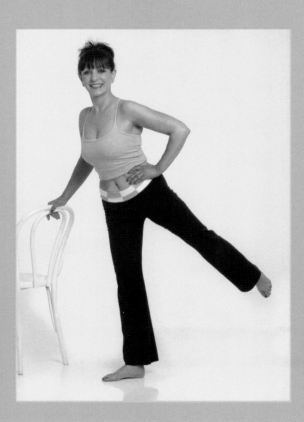

5 Thighs

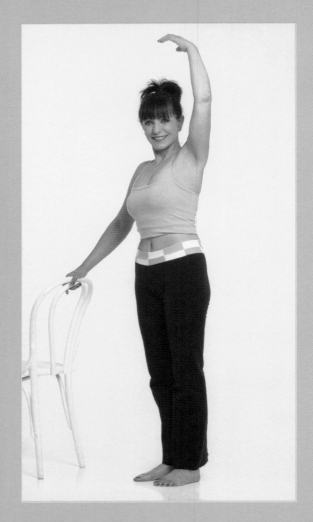

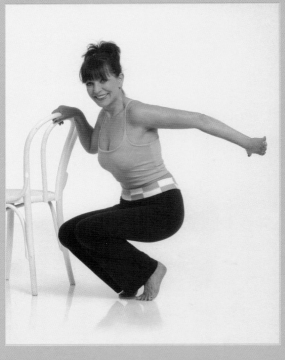

Holding on to the chair as before, make sweeping bends, staying on your toes. Make the action – 'ski-sweep'.

Allow your arms to swing with you. As you come up, raise the arm over your head, then swing down again. Do twelve. If you have knee problems, don't do this one. Your thighs will get enough exercise from climbing stairs or cycling.

6 Chest and Shoulders

a Get on the floor, on all fours.

b Place your hands directly below your shoulders.

c Lower and raise your body, keeping your knees on the floor,
  six to ten times (or many as you can easily manage).

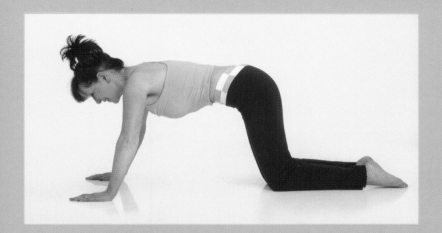

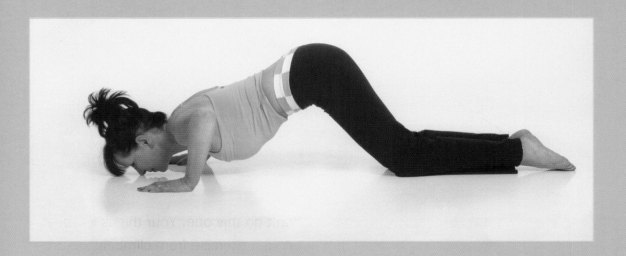

7 Buttocks and Thighs

Now you start combination
movements. This uses the arms,
chest and buttocks.

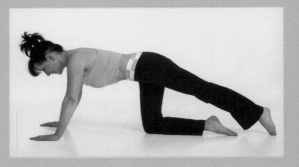

a From the same starting position as for
the press-ups, extend one leg as
shown and tap the toes on the floor.
Press down with your arms and raise
the leg. Repeat ten times.

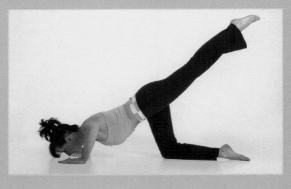

b Now you add on a 'curtsey'. As you
tap your toes on the floor, cross the
leg over the resting leg and press
backwards. This uses your buttock
muscles. Push back up and repeat
ten times.

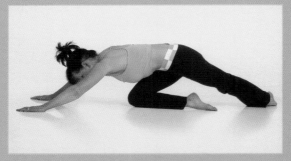

c In the same position, extend the left
leg and draw ten small circles clockwise, then ten anti-clockwise.

d Now change legs and repeat from a.

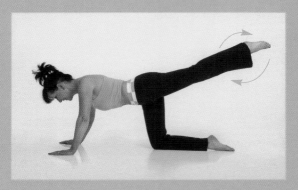

8 Back

a Lie on your front. Place your arms by your sides and keep your legs straight. Slowly lift and lower your back, looking at the floor – do not tip your head or neck back.

b Repeat six times, holding each move for five seconds (a long time!).

c Repeat this move, lifting the legs at the same time. Do six repetitions over one minute.

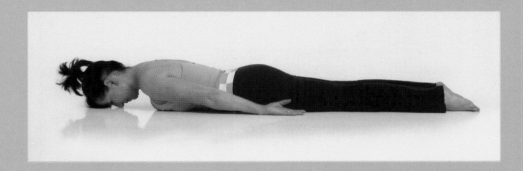

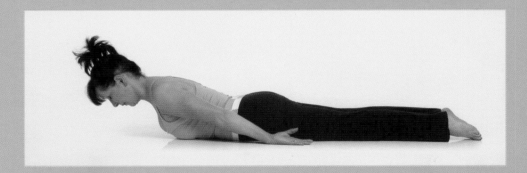

9 Waist

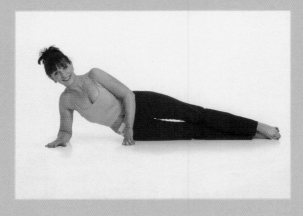

a Lie on your side. Prop your upper body up on your forearm and lift your hips off the floor. Have your legs together on top of each other. Rest your other hand on the floor for support.

b Try to raise and lower your body as shown. Do as many lifts as you can, but six to eight are ideal.

c Take a breather then repeat. Change sides and repeat the whole sequence.

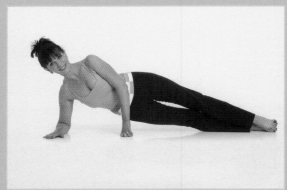

d Sit up, lift the arms and extend them in front of you. Relax back a little, to feel your abdominal muscle engage.

e Lean sideways and reach to tap the floor on left, as shown. Swing over to touch floor on the right.

f Repeat six times slowly on each side. Rest for three seconds, then repeat.

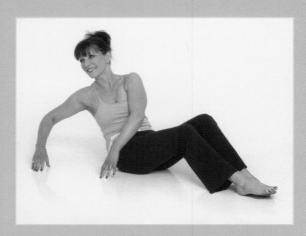

10 Abdomen

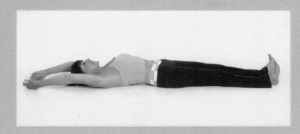

a Lie on your back, extend your legs and flex your feet really hard. Take your arms above your head. Breathe in and then breathe out slowly. As you exhale, press your stomach into your back and feel the floor under the small of your back. Bring your arms overhead.

b Hold this position. The secret is keeping your feet flexed hard. Release and repeat three times in one minute.

c Sit as shown, scooping in your abdominals.

d Breathe in, then out and bring your knees towards your chest, allowing the toes to drop down towards the floor.

e This should be done fast. Use your breath to help you count and do twenty to thirty repetitions in a minute. Rest for ten seconds. Then repeat again.

11 Outer Thighs

Lean onto your side, rest on your elbow
and lift the left leg. Draw small circles,
ten forwards and ten backwards. This
should take a minute. Repeat.

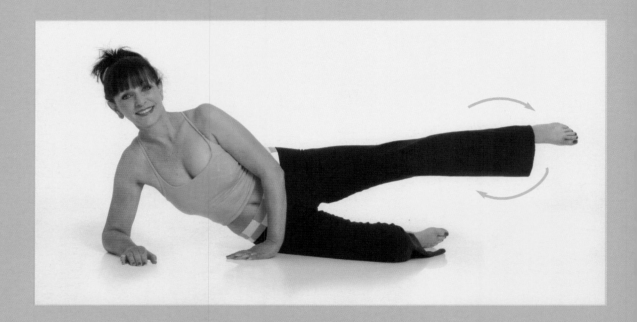

12 Inner Thighs

a Place your top foot on the floor as shown, raise and extend the lower leg.

b Flex the toes hard. Now draw ten tiny circles slowly, clockwise and then anti-clockwise.

c Repeat, this time pointing your toes hard.

Switch onto your other side and repeat exercises 11 and 12 with your other leg.

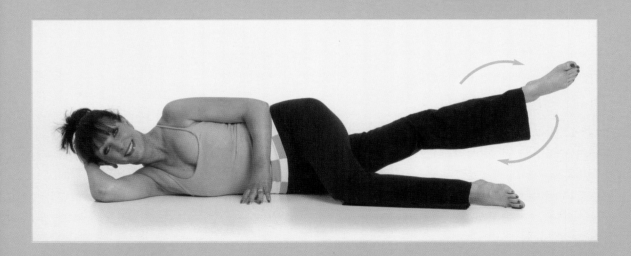

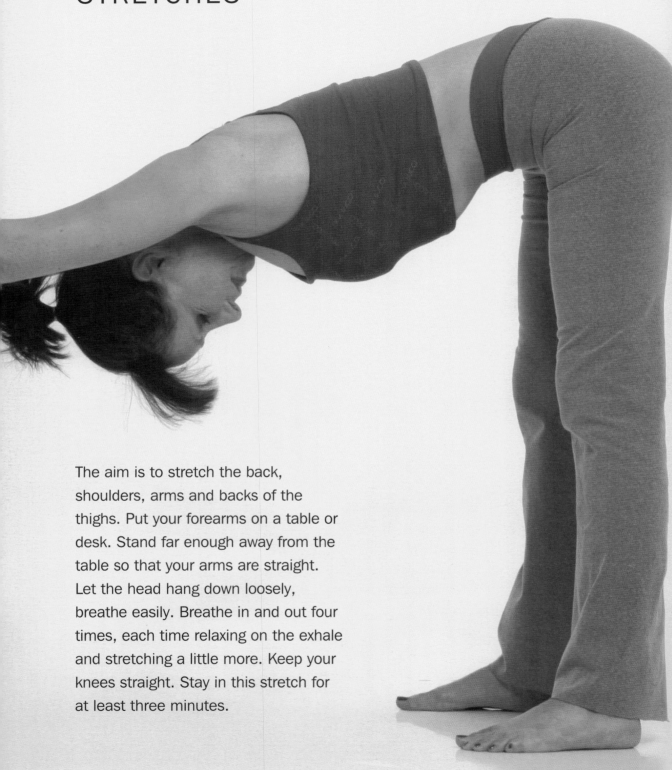

STRETCHES

The aim is to stretch the back, shoulders, arms and backs of the thighs. Put your forearms on a table or desk. Stand far enough away from the table so that your arms are straight. Let the head hang down loosely, breathe easily. Breathe in and out four times, each time relaxing on the exhale and stretching a little more. Keep your knees straight. Stay in this stretch for at least three minutes.

To stretch lower back and backs of legs. This is a straightforward toe-touch, don't worry if you can't manage it – you will eventually and the stretch is equally as effective however far you can manage. Lift your ribcage up and out first, then bring your torso towards the floor on the out breath. Slowly breathe in at the bottom, then try to go further down on the next out breath. To come back up, put your hands on your thighs, exhale, scoop your tummy in and slowly uncurl. Relax for at least three minutes.

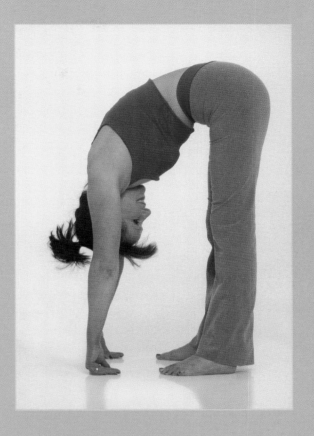

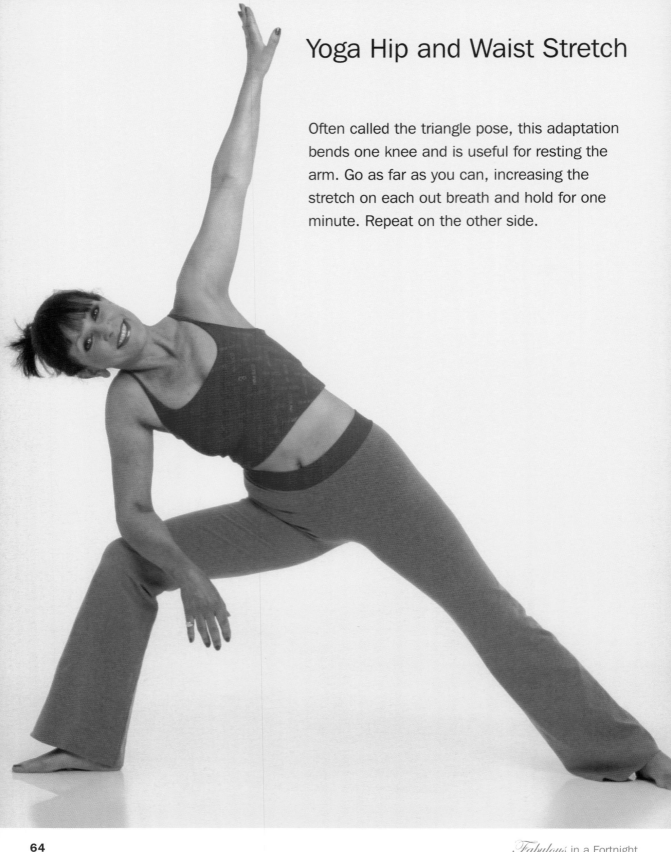

Yoga Hip and Waist Stretch

Often called the triangle pose, this adaptation bends one knee and is useful for resting the arm. Go as far as you can, increasing the stretch on each out breath and hold for one minute. Repeat on the other side.

Hip and Thigh Stretch

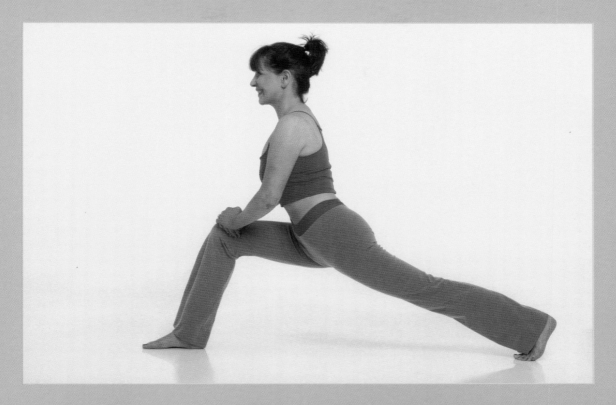

This is hard, but great when you get the hang of it. Take a giant step forwards and relax downwards as shown, making sure your knee is over your toes. Stretch out your back leg and straighten the knee as far as possible. Feel the stretch in your hip. This frees tight hips beautifully. Stretch for one minute.

Tough Thigh Stretch

Moving on, place the back knee on floor, lift your foot and try to reach round with other hand to grab it. Pull it gently towards your buttocks. Hold for one minute. If you find this difficult, do not do it. Repeat both of these stretches on the other leg.

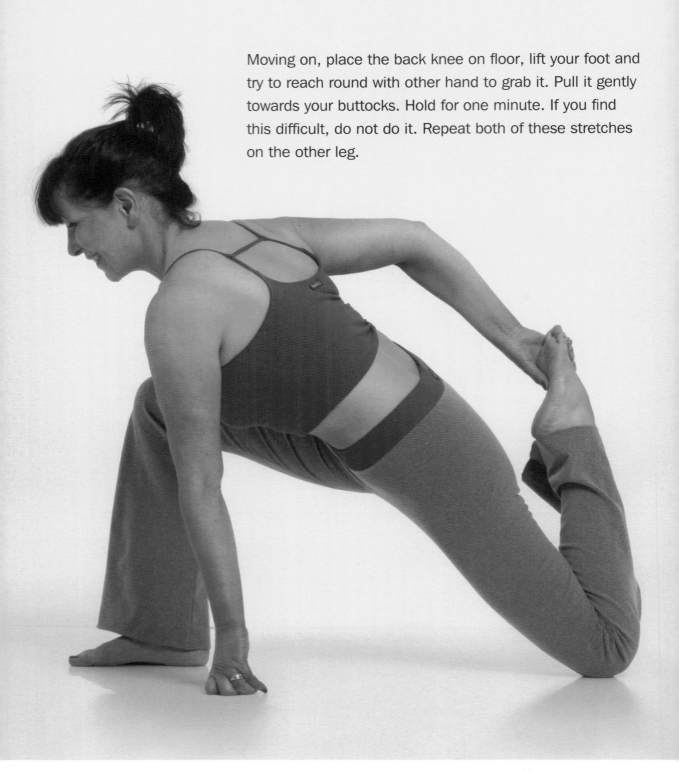

Abdominal Stretch

Important for posture, this also finishes the session on a relaxing note. Lie as flat as possible, stretch the arms overhead and flex your feet hard. Shuffle your hips up and down. Now point the toes hard and hold, increasing the point, for one minute. Flex and repeat the hold, for one minute. Feel the stretch increasing – don't leave it static.

Great! You have finished your Daily Dozen and stretch session. Repeat every day for the full fortnight and every day thereafter.

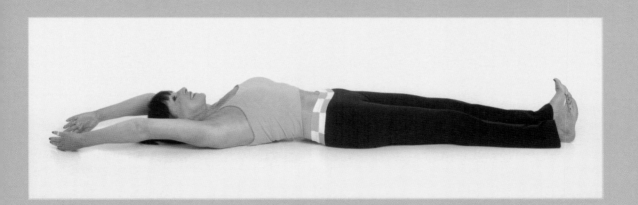

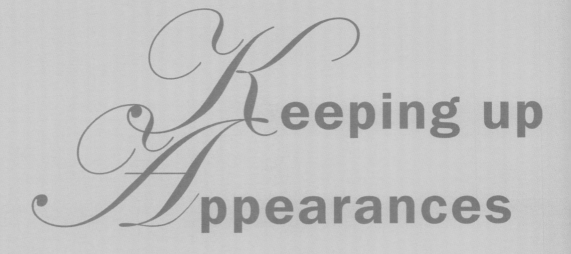

Keeping up Appearances

Your image and what you look like is not the same as the impression you make. Two people wearing jeans and a T-shirt can give very different impressions. If one leans against the wall, smoking and slouching and the other stands with a smile on her face, poised, the effect of the outfits is vastly altered.

You can have your colours done, your style co-ordinated and your image analysed, and these are good places to start if you are thrashing about for inspiration, but it won't necessarily make you a success if you have the wrong image for other reasons. So are such things a waste of time?

Well, yes and no. Everybody goes through a series of style experiments when they're young. The most common mistake is looking and dressing like everybody else just because it is fashionable.

For some people, all the designer labels, correct colours and shapes in the world can't alter the image they give off. Why not use this principle to your advantage? If you haven't got two pennies to rub together and are struggling to look sophisticated on a student grant or income support, you can still portray a classy image.

My late mother was a good example. Widowed young, she struggled to bring us up with just two dresses and a suit to her name. She even mangled the washing wearing high heels. People were more formal back then, but even so. She gave an impression of effortless elegance simply by adding a brooch or string of cheap pearls to an outfit. I'm sure everybody thought those pearls were real. On a tiny budget and two shopping trips a year she looked affluent and sophisticated, rather at odds with the depressing reality.

So how is it done?

People who look classy and elegant portray an understated, sartorially restrained appearance. It might seem politically incorrect to define people in terms of class these days, but looking classy has nothing to do with social status. It is about looking calm and refined. Here are the general guidelines for a classy look:

- simplicity
- good posture
- not too much jewellery
- not using clothes to impress
- clothes sitting comfortably on the body not being particularly over- or underweight
- subtle make-up

Beauty Is an Entire Effect

Looking beautiful and creating an image for yourself depends on tying up all the loose ends. These days, a bit of extra weight is tolerated better than it used to be and you might not feel you have to lose five pounds (2.2 kg) the minute you gain them. But there's a difference between being fat and being what they used to call 'well-upholstered'. The word stout is not the same as fat. Stout suggests you are pretty big but everything is held in. Fat is a lot of bulges. Having said that, some very slender women still manage to spill over their jeans and this is another bad look. The entire effect you portray is what counts, and bulging says 'I don't care'.

Despite the acceptance of larger sizes, I would still advise you to lose weight if you have bulges. We can debate this for ever, but in the final analysis you know if you're bulging and you know how you feel about it. I'd say lose the weight and tone yourself up. A slim figure isn't necessarily a good figure but it's a start. So stand tall, pull yourself in, lift your chest and think: I'm fabulous.

Be Realistic

If you go for a facelift, it won't bring back your errant husband, find you a handsome toyboy or get you invited to more parties. Buying new outfits should carry the same cautionary reminder. If you have your eye on someone and want to beat the opposition, a stunning new dress won't hook him. Well, it might if it's ten inches above the knee and teamed with a pair of thigh-high boots, but that's a different story. In the few years since I first wrote those words, many people have told me that a great outfit makes them feel more confident and in that case, they may succeed in situations where they might otherwise have been self-conscious and timid. I stand corrected. But you still do not have to go out and buy something new, especially if you already have something you know you look good in. Frankly, if you wear a great outfit and feel wrong underneath because you're overweight, your skin is ageing or you are untoned, it won't make a jot of difference.

People Notice What You Look Like

They don't necessarily notice what you are wearing.

If you are showered with compliments every time you wear that green silk suit you bought five years ago, why go out and buy a floaty blue skirt just because it's high fashion? We all need new clothes, but take note of what suits you, build up a comprehensive wardrobe of outfits which incorporate all the best features, and refuse to be swayed by the newest fashion fad unless you're sure it's you. If the outfit has gone totally out of fashion, by all means ditch it. But take note of what works and don't go increasing the national debt just to get noticed, because it won't work. Learn the effects of your favourite outfits and get rid of the ones that don't work.

If In Doubt, Don't!

My own golden rule of thumb for accessories – an extra chain, scarf or bracelet – is that if I have to spend ten minutes doing my utmost to see how they look best, I'm onto a loser. Accessories that are right, look right instantly. If something only looks fantastic if you stand in a pose, forget it. Take it with you to a party by all means. Everybody has carried something they weren't sure of in their handbag, waited to see what everyone else is wearing and then either brought it out or left it hidden. This works the other way round, incidentally. If you are seriously doubting that accessory, or are in two minds about a pair of shoes, make sure your handbag is big enough to take the pair you decided against.

If You Look Good in Something, You'll Always Look Good In It

Most of us have something which we look good in, so if it works, keep wearing it. If an occasion is either unfamiliar or desperately important to you, you won't want to be worrying about how an outfit works. I once scoured the shops in half a dozen cities several hundred miles apart, trying desperately to get a pair of shoes in a certain shade of blue. It seemed important at the time. I found them, wore them to the party which to my dismay was a huge scrum of people, all jostling and elbowing themselves to the bar and shouting to be heard. Needless to say, nothing below my earrings was on view. That was in 1986 and the shoes are still in their box. If only I had put those tortuous efforts and the exorbitant cost into an afternoon relaxing, I would have looked a bit better than I did on the night.

Nobody ever lost her friends just because they'd seen her dress before, and true confidence is having the courage to stay the same. Here's why:

· You'll know how to move, sit, stand and juggle drinks and plates in something you've worn before. A new outfit can be unexpectedly stiff, easily creased, ride up or slide off your shoulders. Only by wearing something will you discover how it works in practice.

· You won't feel self-conscious in it. Being able to forget your outfit is terribly important.

· You'll save time and money, both can be better spent making yourself glamorous in other ways.

I got married in a white suit I'd had for nine years. I had no time to shop and I knew how the suit worked. I could sit, stand, bend, sign the register, pose for photographs and get in and out of cars in it. I knew its little fault of riding up to show the lining if I wasn't careful. I knew the jacket could gape if I didn't undo one button when sitting in a low armchair. Yes, they were faults, but all clothes have their faults. I simply didn't have the time to spend an evening finding out the wearability faults of a whole new wedding outfit.

Try to buy clothes when you don't have anything special in mind and you can devote a day to the search. If you're not desperate you won't mind coming home with nothing, and you'll save money.

Always Carry Spares

It always amazes me when people go out for a whole day taking a silly little handbag with room for no more than a lipstick, comb and the tube fare home. If you ladder your stocking or your zip breaks or you lose the back of your earring, the party's over. The Infamous Disasters section (see page 107) gives real-life stories of disasters which couldn't have been prevented, but which we can all learn from. You don't want to embark on a fun day out carrying a suitcase and looking as though you're off for a fortnight in the Caribbean, but taking a sensible emergency kit with spare tights, plasters, earring backs, hairgrips and slides, wet wipes and powder seems like basic common sense.

Shattering the Illusion

It pays to remember that however much effort you put into your appearance, it's a shame if you spoil the effect with something off-putting. I don't need to mention the obvious, such as foul language or throwing up, but most people have gone down this road and cringe at the memory.

Whether or not you choose to swear like a trooper in public is up to you, but don't be surprised if someone takes exception. It would be a miserable old world if we all went about minding our 'p's and 'q's and never saying anything controversial or shocking, but there's a limit. The limit is when you either upset or offend someone. The limit is definitely reached when you put your career or marriage on the line. If you're among friends who take you as they find you, indiscretions are usually forgiven and forgotten. Remember, though, that some people are friendly but not friends, and have no loyalty to you to keep quiet if they sense a good story at your expense.

Think of the Future

You can't spend your life watching every word in case you feel like standing for parliament in twenty years' time. Worrying about every off-the-cuff remark in case you're drinking with a future employer, or living in fear of a mild profanity in case that gorgeous hunk happens to be the local vicar, is going a bit far. But don't dismiss such cautionary tales out of hand. Depending on where you are on the ladder of life, these things could matter a lot. It takes only a split second to ruin a reputation. A friend who, ten years ago, got drunk at the office Christmas party and lifted her sweater, shouting at the boss, 'What d'you think of that then?' was rewarded with his honest opinion: she wasn't invited to any more parties.

When you are young, it's great to be different from the crowd and it's nice to be noticed and talked about. But people's memories are long when it comes to a major social gaffe and it can be hard to live down. If you liven up some tedious and dull social occasion with your bad behaviour, it could be talked about for years afterwards. Some people even have trouble being taken seriously again. Most problems are fuelled by alcohol, so if you can't hold your drink, don't start. You might get away with a tactless remark, but if you strip naked and seduce your host in front of his wife, you might as well emigrate.

Don't Be Tongue-Tied

It's awful being shy, but knowing that your appearance is spot-on gives you confidence, so work on it. Generally speaking, shy people worry about what to say at parties, thinking that they haven't an opinion. It isn't like that. Ask other people the questions, and remember that we're all human beings who have a lot in common. Let's face it, where would we all be if it wasn't for the good old British weather, stalwart prop of 50 per cent of all conversations?

Keep a Bit Back for Later

Remember if you start at the top, the only place to go is down. If you tell your best jokes, dazzle everyone with your stunning beauty, fantastic dancing and the amazing story of your life, you won't have the same appeal when you run into someone in the supermarket on a wet Saturday afternoon. It isn't so bad if you're in familiar company and everyone knows you, but don't go the whole hog among strangers. I've spoken to hundreds of men about what shattered their illusions about someone or put them off. 'Not keeping a bit back for another time' was high on the list.

Mystery is important. However extrovert you are, however effervescent and bubbly and full of life – keep a bit back for next time.

Never Underestimate Scarcity Value

When there's rumour of an imminent shortage of something, everyone wants it. The same goes for people. However, scarcity value shouldn't be confused with playing hard to get, that tedious game which wins you no friends and gets you a reputation as haughty and hard work. Scarcity value is a genuine incentive to men to try that bit harder to win you.

The trick is to be bright, breezy and not too available. You don't need to go as far as I once did and write yourself a dozen unlikely invitation cards to prop up on your mantelpiece the minute Mr Wonderful drops by. I even got my friends to call me intermittently between six and half past, so he would think I had dozens of other boyfriends. Well, who doesn't? Being unavailable means you can't get a babysitter, your exams are looming or you can't get a night off work. The old hair-washing routine always worked a treat, because when a man thinks your hair is more important than him, he'll try even harder. And when you do say yes, he won't take you for granted.

Tips To Improve Your Image

This is so easy; you'll wonder why you wasted all that money on clothes.

- Smile as much as you can. Smile the minute you enter a room, however nervous you are. If it doesn't come naturally, practise at home in your bedroom until you get it right. Borrow a camcorder if possible and watch yourself. Coming into a room with a worried expression shows you up as self-conscious and unsure.
- Stand up straight (see 'What about body language?', page 75).
- Listen attentively to the person you're speaking to. However tempted you may be, don't look over their shoulder, even for a second.
- Remember people's names. They'll be flattered and like you all the more.
- Look interested. People aren't looking to you to entertain them, but by appearing interested in others you will draw them to you. However daunting someone seems, perhaps as a captain of industry or the third richest person in England or a TV soap-opera star, they still have home lives like the rest of us. An old college friend of mine who became a household name on television once lamented that at parties people never asked about her work, or commented on it. Remember, most people like being asked questions about their lives.
- Don't fiddle with your handbag, jewellery or hair. It is intensely distracting to the other person who might be having trouble relaxing themselves, it looks self-conscious and nervous and you might come across as troubled or hard work.
- If you receive a compliment, accept it with a 'Thank you'. Far too many women devalue a compliment by arguing against it.
- Work on your voice if you're worried about it. Many an illusion is shattered the minute someone opens his or her mouth.

What Is Your Face Saying?

If people keep on telling you to 'Cheer-up – it might never happen', take it seriously. You might be having a whale of a time or be concentrating on the finer points of someone's story, but what is your face saying?

Nobody wants to get stuck with someone who looks like hard work, and if they sense they're going to be treated to an hour's lecture on the unfairness of the child-support system or the dog's life your ex-husband gave you, they're not even going to start.

Study yourself. Make a pleasant face, which is 'lifted', without actually smiling. Think of something nice which brings a slight sparkle to your eyes, lift your eyebrows just a little. Think lift. Remember how it feels, and while you are training yourself, put a mirror nearby in which you can keep checking.

All these things – your voice, your expression and your posture – are matters of habit. If you can get into bad habits you can also get into good ones. Remember that you can become whatever you want to become, and it doesn't take much effort to really make something of yourself. All this effort, all the exercise and dieting, new clothes and hair conditioning will be money down the drain if you forget to smile and look bright and cheerful. You can't help feeling miserable if life is tough, but you don't have to look it.

You *can* look fabulous, you *can* draw admiring glances and have people talking about you if you believe in yourself. It doesn't take money, it takes confidence. Don't get caught out slouching, chewing, or with your stomach hanging slackly. Most important, never be caught out looking sour.

Practise how you look. Stand tall. Smile.

Your Voice

If you have a tape recorder, it isn't a bad idea to record your voice. Most of us have done this at some time in our lives, and I don't know anyone who wasn't horrified. In truth, we don't usually sound as bad as we fear, but if you have a habit of speaking too quickly, too loudly, or cutting off the ends of your words, it doesn't hurt to be aware of it because it can give the wrong impression. You might think it's too late to do anything about your voice, but a conscious effort to speak a little more slowly, to pitch your voice down a bit or to speak more clearly can easily be learned in a few days. Do listen to yourself speaking, or ask a friend for an honest opinion.

What About Body Language?

It's time you thought about posture. No matter what you put on your back or how much money you spend beautifying yourself, a hunched, slouched appearance destroys the whole effect.

In case you think that a straight back is all right for formal occasions but not so appropriate at casual events, I'm going to show you that you can look relaxed and confident even when sitting on a sofa in a pair of jeans and a sweater. Confidence is all about good posture, so let's start with the basics.

Place a large, but not too heavy, book on your head. Move it about until it feels comfortable and won't fall off.

Walk around the room, remembering to relax your shoulders. Look at yourself in a full-length mirror. You might feel your chin is too high and you are looking up. You aren't. Your chest might also feel thrust out. It isn't. Walk around the room again and remember what it feels like.

Practise this posture for a few minutes twice a day until you get used to it. Good posture is youthful. Good posture spells confidence. Practice makes perfect.

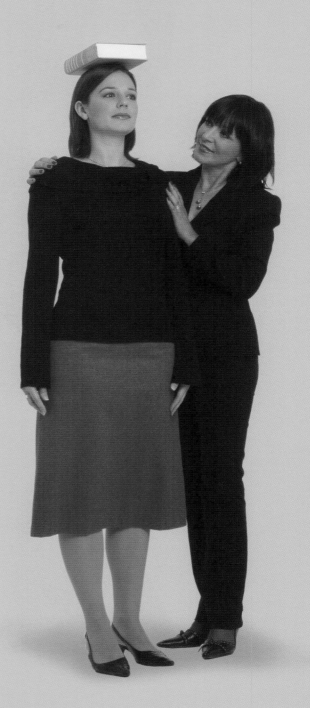

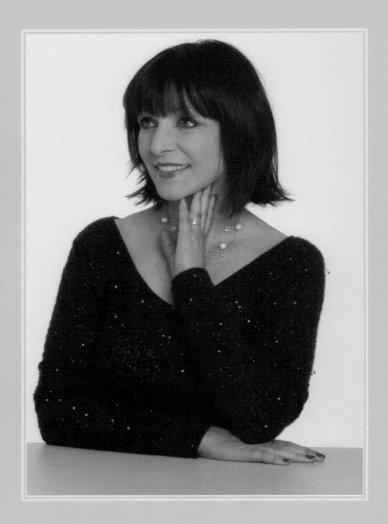

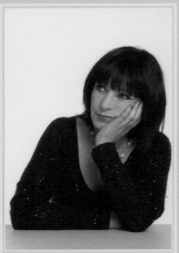

This sitting position (inset below), is very common, especially when it's late and you are tired, or you've had a bit too much to drink!

The picture above may look a little formal, but you are still leaning on the table in a relaxed way. By keeping your back straight you look alert and interested in what people have to say, all of which gains you bonus points. It is especially important to maintain an alert bearing if you are attending a company or business function, because even if your attitude and performance are not actually being assessed, it might be unconsciously noted that your professional bearing can slip, or was not natural.

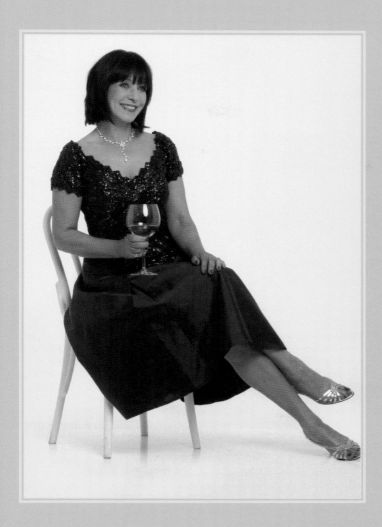

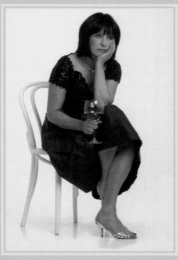

If you're sitting for hours at a party and are absorbed by the conversation, it's easy to adopt the wrong posture. By raising your upper chest, the effect is far more pleasing. Again, you can look relaxed but not sloppy. Note that the neck is lengthened, not hunched.

In the picture opposite, by cupping your chin in this way you are not only forcing your mouth into an unattractive line, you are distorting your cheek and probably smudging your make-up. The hunched position will also leave your neck and shoulders tense. Sit up straight, bring your chair nearer to the table, and feel the lower part of your back in contact with it. By practising now, sitting up straight will come to you naturally in the future.

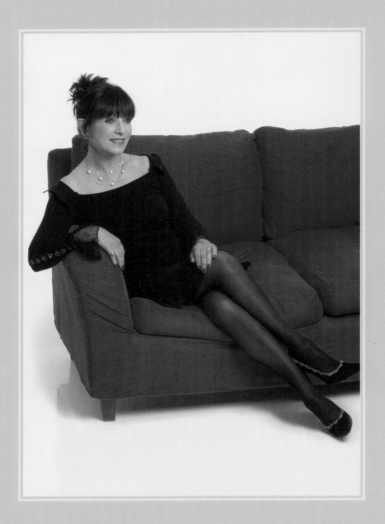

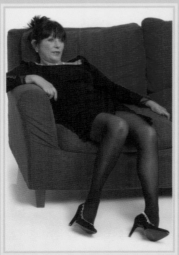

It's late and you're tired. Maybe a little too much to drink and eat. You get absorbed in the conversation or just find it hard to keep your eyes open. It's easy to undo all the hard work of getting ready and suddenly your double chin and underwear are on show for everyone to see!

Get a grip and sit up. You can still relax by placing your bottom up against the back of the sofa for support. Keep your legs together and crossed to the side for a nice long line and don't collapse your ribcage. You'll be home soon, but for the moment don't forget you're still on show!

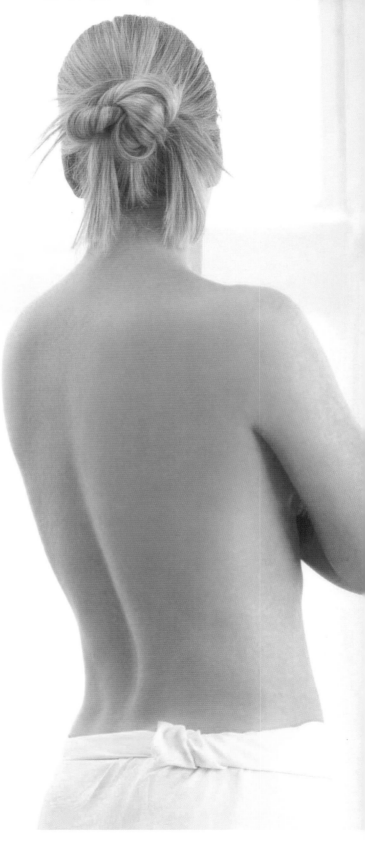

Beauty

Take an honest look at yourself. Most of us are pretty negative about our looks. We insist there's nothing we're happy with, but is that really true? Let's start with your weight.

Stand in front of a full-length mirror wearing underwear and a well-fitting T-shirt or vest. Looking at yourself, where does your body carry extra weight? You might feel heavy, but where does the weight actually settle? Everyone knows her own body from how her clothes fit, but it never ceases to amaze me that people still judge their figures by what the scales say. You must forget this! Your weight doesn't tell you what you look like.

Hold a hand-mirror and take a look at your back view. Does your bottom really need to be smaller, or is it simply lacking tone?

Your Back

I suggested wearing a close-fitting T-shirt or vest because it shows up the state of your back. Many women put on weight from the top down, and fat is often stored on the upper back and under the arms. We all have sheets of powerful muscles which allow us to do a whole range of arm movements, but when these muscles get slack they can also manifest themselves as a flabby back which causes unsightly bulges.

Bras highlight the problem because their very nature means they have to fit closely. If you have a lot of over- and under-hang, don't wear tight tops.

Your Front

The same goes for your front view. If your top is going to be revealing, you need a smooth line underneath – so no lace or bows on your bra. Choose one which encases your whole breast, and definitely don't wear balcony or uplift bras under bodies or T-shirts. They emphasize any spare breast flesh which might not be in the first flush of youth!

The only women who have genuinely pert, uplifted breasts are about fifteen. Due to the predominance of TV programmes portraying beach loads of silky siliconed beauties, and the fact that breasts are always covered, lifted or squeezed into shapes Mother Nature never intended, we should be forgiven for thinking we're falling short if ours are droopy (or 'soft', as a high-class corsetière put it rather delicately), small or mismatching. Your bosom is there, so you might as well make the most of it, and a good bustline is a sign of youthfulness.

If you're small, don't make the mistake of thinking that you don't need support; always wear a good bra.

Keep Reappraising the Situation

It's extraordinary that some women buy the same bra size for as long as forty years. Even if your weight has not fluctuated, there's a huge difference between the ages of twenty-five and forty-five in breast terms, and even if your measurement is the same, the way your flesh has settled could be very different. Remember that the measurement round your bust takes in a lot more than just breast tissue. It includes your back and under your arms, so check every two or three years that your cup size hasn't altered.

Having a well-fitted bra makes a world of difference to your outline and figure.

Your Legs

Good legs are classy and an essential part of looking fabulous. What are yours like?

During the past fifteen years or so, there's been a vague feeling of political incorrectness in the suggestion that men like to look at a pretty leg in a flattering shoe. Grunge fashions, clumpy boots and long skirts have all contributed to women losing interest in their lower legs, though for some reason the spotlight has swung upwards to our thighs. Today's exercise excesses have developed muscular calves and thick ankles, not to mention large thighs, and I think it's a shame that so little interest is shown in the part of the legs everyone sees.

If you have problem legs, or even if you don't, here is what you must do:

1 Follow the foot and leg exercises in the exercise section, every day.
2 Keep your legs permanently hair-free and moisturized.
3 Keep your feet immaculate – it will give you a psychological boost.
4 Reduce puffy ankles by drinking two extra pints of water a day – strange though it may seem, water helps reduce fluid retention.
5 Wear dark-coloured tights, and wear tights and shoes of the same tone – this makes your legs look longer and slimmer.

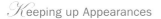

Your Feet

Feet can be a sadly neglected area, but they are not something you can afford to miss. In a crowded life, it's enough that we have to be faced with even the simplest daily beauty routine, never mind adding our hands and feet to the list! It's all too easy to shove on a pair of shoes so it's a case of 'out of sight and out of mind'.

However, rather like the old chestnut about wearing clean knickers in case you have an accident, neglecting your feet in the hope that nobody will ever see them is fraught with hazards. I once worked with a glamorous and immaculate woman, known and admired for her designer suits, expensive haircuts and lacquered nails. One hot summer's afternoon she arrived for a meeting in the usual eye-catching ensemble but, unfortunately, she was also wearing open-toed sandals and had bare legs. At one stage in the proceedings I looked down at the floor and was alarmed to see a set of gnarled, yellow toes poking out from her shoes and two appallingly dry and cracked heels. I simply couldn't believe my eyes, and neither could anyone else once I'd drawn their attention to it! This wasn't just an oversight, it was long-term, serious neglect and, what's more, it marked her out for ever with her gleeful colleagues as a person who was all 'top show'. It was years ago, but whenever we get together and her name comes up, all we can remember about her is her dreadful feet!

Don't get caught out. A weekly home pedicure should take no more than twenty minutes.

Your Hands and Nails

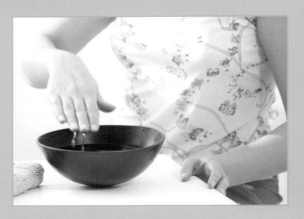

It's no good having long, strong nails if they look like something you'd find on the end of a parrot's claws. Long nails are fine if they look as if you have deliberately cultivated them that way. They're not fine when they look as if they're long only because you can't get round to cutting them. Ragged and dry cuticles are also signs of neglect, and the fabulous woman doesn't neglect anything.

On the other hand, short nails can be either a disaster or chic, depending on the state of them. If they look short because you like them that way, you take care of them and they shine healthily, that's great. If they are short because you've either bitten them down to the quick or been laying the patio with your bare hands, not so great. At the end of the day, long or short, it doesn't matter as long as your hands look cared for.

Your Face

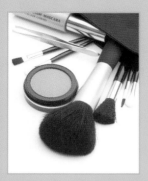

Your face gets some pretty rough treatment, and it gets all the criticism as well. You can't change what you've got in the next fortnight, but you can make a huge difference to the way you look.

· Do your eyebrows need plucking?
· Does your upper lip need waxing or depilation?
· Have you many spots?
· Is your complexion dull and lifeless?
· Is your skin grimy? (Test with cotton wool soaked in a skin freshener.)
· Does your make-up need an overhaul?

Your Neck

It's extraordinary how a woman's neck can let her down. We pay attention to our faces and hair and the neck somehow gets forgotten.

If you're young, and by that I mean anything from sixteen to about twenty, I urge you with all my heart to start taking care of your neck. By the time you're thirty or forty, if your neck's gone, you can't do a thing about it. What do I mean by 'gone': rings round the neck, slack skin which resembles a turkey's, lots of spots and freckles. I know it's not too palatable to talk about it, but this is what anyone's neck ends up like when a) they've spent a life sunbathing; b) they haven't moisturized their neck; and c) they haven't kept their neck clean.

The same applies to your upper chest and shoulders. The area above your bustline gets exposure when you wear low-cut dresses and tops, swimsuits, T-shirts and so on. Start when you're a teenager: put on a nightly covering of a good moisturizer, and clean it off in the morning. In fact, keep your neck and chest as scrupulously clean as you would your face.

If you have neglected your neck, don't worry. We all have something we're a bit sensitive about, and you can make sure you minimize further damage by starting to cleanse and moisturize.

Your Hair

The fabulous woman's hair always looks just right. It doesn't matter if you've been struggling through a gale-force wind or caught in a shower, once you've got the right style and condition, you can take such minor disasters in your stride.

The basis of lovely hair is a good cut. Does yours need a trim? Split ends and straggly long hair are instant signs of hair which has been forgotten about, and that says a lot about you. Although you're doing most things yourself in the next fortnight, you need a professional cut, so make an appointment. You don't want to leave it too late and find you can't get in.

However, a complete re-style or major cut is not a good idea right now, unless you are positive that it will make you feel better, or if you have had the style before and want to go back to it. If you are getting ready for a major event it could be disastrous, because you might not be able to think of anything else. Remember too that a completely different hairstyle will throw your clothes choices out of balance. Unless you really want to go out and buy a lot of new clothes, stick with what you've got until a time when the stakes aren't so high.

The Fabulous in a Fortnight Programme

The fabulous in a fortnight programme

is your full schedule of diet, exercise and

beauty. Think of it like a training course:

you will emerge at the end of two weeks

having learnt a great deal about yourself,

not least that you can make a lot of

headway and really transform yourself

when you concentrate your efforts.

If you are like most people, you'll want a straightforward menu plan for fourteen days that you simply pin up and follow. You can go away, buy the ingredients and get on with something else. Everybody has better things to do, but thinking about meals has to take priority in the long run or you might land in the same place you were before. So try to get the hang of it, pick from the lists of meals (pages 86 to 98) or why not write out your own charts? Lots of people find this a better option, keeping the lists of anytime food in the middle column and writing their own protein or starch meals in the appropriate columns. It's quite a good game for children to play, too, as you plan meals together and get them to write their choices in the appropriate column.

As always, these meals are ideas. You don't have to follow them to the letter, except to separate protein and starch meals and eat a starch meal for dinner during the first fortnight.

I am told by shift-workers, night workers, part-timers and others with unsocial patterns, that the terms breakfast, lunch and dinner annoy them intensely. I can see why. I have therefore numbered the meals, and you can shift them about to suit yourself. For example, if you are working nights, finish at 7 a.m. and are in bed by 8 a.m., you should eat a starch meal on your last break. This is the third meal. You would have your second meal in the middle of your shift, which could be midnight. Play around with this, but I guarantee it will work. Difficult working patterns should never be an excuse for weight gain and this diet works well with any lifestyle. As always, experiment!

I have given page references for those dishes for which I have given recipes. An asterisk against a particular meal denotes it is very low in calories.

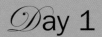ay 1

FIRST MEAL
Mixed fruit salad with 2tbs plain yoghurt
or
2 whole oranges, 1 grapefruit, segmented*

SECOND MEAL
Herb or mushroom omelette with salad
or
Smoked Salmon and Avocado Salad page 129

THIRD MEAL
Mushroom Medley Risotto page 122
or
Jacket potato, baked beans and salad
or
Cannelloni Stuffed with Spinach and Almonds
page 123*

SUPPER
Poached Stuffed Peach page 138
Crème fraiche or yoghurt with pineapple,
grape and orange fruit salad

Tip

Hands, beauty-wise, rank right after
face and voice. Make your hands work
for you, not against you.

1 Be careful about a lot of hand-
   waggling. If you find you are using
   gestures instead of words, stop
   yourself. We all know that gesture
   when you are searching for a word
   and can't find it – wild shaking as you
   search your memory. It is far more
   soothing for your audience and your
   own nerves if you practise sitting with
   your hands folded in your lap or, if
   standing, clasped gently at hip level or
   even hanging straight by your sides.

2 Wear gloves where possible. They
   protect your skin and keep hands
   wrinkle-free.

3 If your wrists are thick, chunky
   watches and bracelets only make
   them seem thicker. Wear thin,
   slightly dangling single-strand
   bracelets.

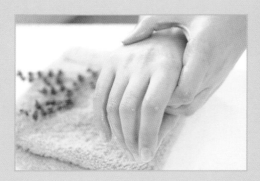

Day 2

FIRST MEAL
Strawberry, raspberry and mango smoothie
with 2tbs yoghurt
or
Cottage cheese and fruit platter. Cut the top
off a large orange, scoop out the flesh and fill
the inside with low-fat cottage cheese. Put on
a plate and surround with sliced apple, pear,
10 grapes, strawberries, raspberries, etc.
or
2 whole oranges, 1 grapefruit, segmented*

SECOND MEAL
Two lean beef burgers* (preferably home-
made) with sweetcorn, peas and a colourful
mixed salad
or
Oriental Tofu and Pine Nut Salad page 132*
or
Skinny Chicken and Garden Grill page 117

THIRD MEAL
Pasta Primavera page 120*
or
Cream cheese and grape baguette, extra
salad
or
Wild rice and pecan nut salad*
Portion Rice Pudding page 137

SUPPER
Mixed fruit salad
or
3 pieces of fresh fruit

Tip

It doesn't hurt to practise your walk –
for any occasion. Indeed, I have known
people deliberately find themselves a
new walk, in the same way they might
find a new hairstyle.
It's a fantastic idea.

1 Pick a place where you can walk at
   least twenty paces in a straight line.
2 Let your arms hang and place your
   palms on your thighs.
3 Saunter forwards, allowing your hips
   to take the lead.
4 Hold in your tummy and lift your
   ribcage up off your waist.
5 Practise crossing each foot over the
   other so your walk is almost pigeon-
   toed. This is an exaggeration, but
   you need to overdo it in order to
   perfect it. See what this feels like.
   If it helps, imagine you are a model
   and copy their walk. It will look
   completely normal.
6 Practise your walk every day.

$\mathcal{D}$ay 3

FIRST MEAL
Fresh fruit salad, 2tbs fromage frais (optional)
or
2 whole oranges, 1 grapefruit, segmented*

SECOND MEAL
Tuna or cold salmon salad
or
Bacon and Walnut Salad page 130
or
Two slices cold chicken and salad with orange
vinaigrette dressing*

THIRD MEAL
Vegetable curry with rice and salad
or
Two slices wholegrain toast topped with
tomatoes
or
2 cakes of bubble and squeak (potato,
cabbage and onion)
Small pot yoghurt*

SUPPER
Winter Fruit Salad page 138
with fromage frais

Tip

Why do we start every morning with a
wake-up stretch by a window? Doesn't
it seem a bit pointless?

Well, a wake-up stretch does exactly
that – it wakes you up. When we're
sleeping, our breathing is shallow,
we're scrunched up into a ball more
often than not, or we've been in one
position for several hours. Stretching
out feels good and the deep intake of
oxygen into the bloodstream revives our
sluggish system and makes us feel
much fresher and more wide awake,
more quickly. So never ignore your
wake-up stretch. Your muscles need it,
and your circulation will also benefit.

Are you doing your exercises? Even if
they are difficult, most people can do at
least one movement. Standing on one
leg and swinging the other is easy for
most people. It wakes up your hips and
reminds your fat stores that they won't
find a quiet place to settle down here!

Once you have mastered one
exercise, you will certainly master the
others. Take your time.

Fabulous in a Fortnight

Day 4

FIRST MEAL
Strawberry, raspberry and mango smoothie
with 2tbs yoghurt
or
Banana, sliced with mango chunks and 2tbs
yoghurt

SECOND MEAL
Avocado and prawns on salad with
vinaigrette dressing
or
Cottage cheese and mixed fruit platter*
or
2 slices roast lamb or beef, carrots,
broccoli and peas

THIRD MEAL
Vegetable chilli with 4tbs rice
or
Penne pasta with crème fraiche and toasted
pine nuts served with spinach
or
Noodles with sesame oil, peas and broad
beans, 1tbs pine nuts, toasted*
Plain yoghurt (optional)

SUPPER
Stewed blackberry and apple with crème
fraiche
or
Stewed fresh or tinned plums and fromage
frais or crème fraiche

Tip

Switch heels at least once every day.
A steady diet of low or high heels
makes some of your muscles lazy, and
over-develops others. If you are in flat
shoes all day, wear something high if
only for an hour when you get home,
and vice versa.

Fleshy knees can be cured by doing
leg circles from the knee downwards.
You can do this when relaxing
anywhere or under the desk at work!

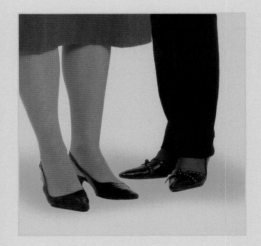

ay 5

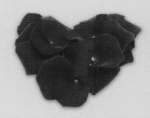

FIRST MEAL
Banana, papaya and mango smoothie with yoghurt

or

2 whole oranges, 1 grapefruit, segmented*

or

Fresh fruit salad with 2tbs yoghurt

SECOND MEAL
Egg mayonnaise salad

or

Plain ham salad*

or

Beef stroganoff made with cream, mushrooms and onions with salad or fresh steamed vegetables

THIRD MEAL
Linguini in Creamy Watercress Sauce page 120

or

Vegetable quiche with French beans and potatoes

or

168g baked potato and salad including carrot and sweetcorn*

SUPPER
Mixed exotic fruit salad with mango, pineapple, grapes and kiwi fruit

Tip

Perfume is the accessory that pulls good looks together. The life expectancy of most good perfumes is four hours. Take some with you if you are going to be out all day.

Never make the mistake of spraying your hair with perfume. The scent mingles with your own hair oils and can change completely. You should spray or dab perfume into your palm, then pat once on the top of your head. It is heaven for any man you dance with or get into a clinch with.

Best perfume sites –

- backs of knees
- inside elbows
- nape of neck
- décolletage
- wrists

Day 6

FIRST MEAL
2 whole oranges, 1 grapefruit, segmented*
or
Large latte coffee with a bowl of grapefruit segments

SECOND MEAL
Spiced Lamb Salad with Mango Dressing page 128*
or
Spanish omelette (made with 2 whole eggs and 4 whites) and salad with sweetcorn (do not have this if you had eggs for breakfast)
or
Cottage pie made with mince, onions, mushrooms, parsnip mash and fresh greens

THIRD MEAL
Vegetable curry with salad
or
Half a vegetable pizza with olives and a mixed colourful salad including peppers and grated carrot
Rice Pudding page 137

SUPPER
2 pieces of fruit
or
Mixed fruit salad

Tip

Have you rehearsed yet?

Just as any good wedding would warrant a decent run-through of procedures, if your special occasion is important you'll need to rehearse.

Always check you can handle all the bits and pieces you'll be carrying. For example, you might find yourself at an outdoor event on a windy day and be caught having to use one hand to hold onto your hat, leaving the other for your handbag, glass and to manage your hemline!

There is nothing worse than having to spend an entire day lugging around a bag that feels like a suitcase or trying to hold shut a button that won't do its job. It is so tedious to be checking your cleavage all the time in case your bra is showing yet again.

Don't just prance in front of a mirror – if necessary, wear your clothes to something else as a dummy run. A good rehearsal is never wasted.

Day 7

FIRST MEAL
2 whole oranges, 1 grapefruit, segmented*
or
Strawberry, raspberry and mango smoothie
with 2tbs yoghurt

SECOND MEAL
Chicken with Watermelon and Hazelnut Salad
with Raspberry Vinaigrette page 113*
or
Any roast meat or poultry, green vegetables
and carrots, no potatoes
or
Lamb moussaka made with onions and
tomatoes, aubergines and grated cheese

THIRD MEAL
Jacket potato with salad and sweetcorn
or
Linguini in Creamy Watercress Sauce page 120
or
Home-made pizza-ciabatta (half a ciabatta)
with olives, tomatoes, Parmesan, capers and
goat's cheese, grilled and drizzled with olive oil

SUPPER
Fromage frais with fruit compote (available
in jars in good supermarkets), plus one apple
chopped into quarters
or
Small pot plain bio-yoghurt with raisins,
chopped walnuts and an apple

Tip

A lovely smile is one of your best assets.
However much time you spend on your
looks, however many conditioning
treatments you've had or how ravishing
your body, a hard face ruins it all. Some
people actually cultivate an aloofness which
masquerades as 'cool'.

In the real world we all need to make
friends and influence people. It pays to look
approachable. People find it hard to pluck
up courage to speak to someone new
unless they've been introduced, and paving
the way by looking pleasant is helping you
as much as it is helping them.

It works in all walks of life. Nobody
wants to employ someone who looks as
if they're going to go off the deep end at
every small criticism. If you're new in a
neighbourhood, people will look at you first
to gauge whether you're likely to welcome a
knock on the door. Any man who's thinking
of asking you out for a drink will consider
initially if it's going to be worth his while
even trying and, however glamorous you
look, a hard, unfriendly face isn't likely to
encourage him. It's difficult to put on a
cheerful face if you've got all the troubles
of the world on your shoulders, but looking
pleasant is as easy as looking miserable,
so practise your smile. You're building up
your assets as you go along, and most of
these come for free.

Day 8

FIRST MEAL
2 whole oranges, 1 grapefruit, segmented*
or
Pot of yoghurt with one grated apple and
a sliced banana

SECOND MEAL
2 slices smoked salmon with capers, crème
fraiche and salad *
or
Lemon Paprika Chicken with Walnuts
page 111*
or
Roast cod with broad beans and pureed peas

THIRD MEAL
Spiced Vegetable Triangles page 127,
with either green vegetables, carrot batons
or
Vegetable stir-fry with soy sauce and a small
jacket potato*
or
Nuts and Bolts Pasta Salad page 122*
Stewed blackberry and apple or fruit of your
choice (tinned will do)

SUPPER
Winter Fruit Salad page 138
with fromage frais*

Tip

How's the diet going? Have you found it
hard or not so bad?

When you're young it's easy to think
you've all the time in the world. A few
months' lapse, gaining a few pounds,
getting out of condition and a bit flabby . . .
there's always the New Year, or next week.

You're crazy to let your best years slip
away like that. You really are young only
once. While you've got what it takes, take
all you can. I'm not saying it's too late in
middle age, far from it. But youth is there
to be enjoyed, and knowing you look your
best will not only help you get the best out
of life but release a whole area of stress.
There's a huge amount of competition out
there. You've only got six more days of the
initial programme and who knows what the
new you will achieve?
Go for it!!

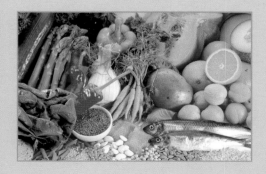

Day 9

FIRST MEAL
2 whole oranges, 1 grapefruit, segmented*
or
Strawberry, raspberry and mango smoothie
with 2tbs yoghurt

SECOND MEAL
Salade Niçoise page 131
or
Steak and salad
or
Lamb moussaka with onions and tomatoes,
aubergines and grated cheese

THIRD MEAL
Jacket potato with salad and sweetcorn
or
Vegetable Chilli page 124
or
Two rounds of wholemeal salad sandwiches

SUPPER
Fromage frais with fruit compote (available
in jars in good supermarkets), plus one apple
chopped into quarters
or
Small pot plain bio-yoghurt with raisins,
chopped walnuts and an apple

Tip

Every woman cannot be a beauty. But
you can delight everyone who sees you.
Every woman has one exceptional
aspect, whether it is her hair colour or
texture, her immaculate attention to
detail or something as everyday as a
perfect manicure.

  You might have a wonderful bearing,
poise or look deeply influential. You
could simply smell delicious, something
that costs little and takes no time.
Indeed, these little touches, like your
scent, soft skin or beautiful posture
could be your quickest way of creating
a wonderful impression.

Day 10

FIRST MEAL
2 whole oranges, 1 grapefruit, segmented*
or
Fresh fruit salad with strawberries,
raspberries, half an apple, sliced mango and
a few grapes

SECOND MEAL
Avocado and prawns on salad with
vinaigrette dressing
or
Scallop and Bacon Provençale page 116*
or
Cold chicken breast, cubed, 2 sliced
tomatoes, cucumber but no dressing*

THIRD MEAL
1 slice spinach and tomato or asparagus
quiche with green vegetables and 2 new potatoes
or
Layered vegetable pie with mashed potato
or
Carrot or spinach soup with one wholemeal
roll*

SUPPER
Poached Pear, served with yoghurt page 137

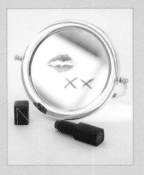

Tip

It is time to go through the boring but
essential checks for your final look.

1 Put on your outfit and check for
   underwear showing.
2 Check for visible panty lines.
3 Check for bra bulge.
4 If you are wearing stockings, double-
   check that you can sit down in your
   skirt and not have to keep tugging at
   your hem to hide the welts.
5 Don't rely on a jacket to hide a faulty
   dress or blouse underneath. The
   weather might change and be
   unexpectedly hot and you may long
   to take it off, except you can't. You
   might spill something and have to
   remove it. If all is not in order
   underneath you could be severely
   embarrassed.

Day 11

FIRST MEAL
2 whole oranges, 1 grapefruit, segmented*
or
2tbs cottage cheese with half a papaya,
sliced, banana and 6 grapes

SECOND MEAL
Seafood salad*
or
2 scrambled eggs, 2 rashers lean bacon,
tomatoes and mushrooms
or
Avocado and pine nut salad

THIRD MEAL
Small vegetable pizza with a colourful mixed
salad
or
3 roast potatoes, Brussels sprouts, carrots,
peas and gravy with mint sauce or horseradish*
or
Cannelloni Stuffed with Spinach and Almonds
page 123

SUPPER
Mixed fruit salad with 1 apple, 1 pear and 10
grapes
or
Small tin fruit salad
or
Baked Apple and Fromage Frais page 136

Tip

A well-proportioned chest is one of the
most important aspects of your look.
Have you had your bra size checked
recently?

Even if your weight and dress size
have not altered, I can guarantee that
your cup size will have changed several
times over the years. Fat is lost from
your boobs as you get older. Don't
replace it, but develop the underlying
chest muscles. They provide nature's
own bra. Here is an exercise you must
do every day from now on:

Sit on a chair, feet flat. Grab each
wrist. Now move as if you were pushing
up the sleeves of your blouse, but keep
the hands in the same place. Squeeze
and hold. You will feel those muscles
'jump' slightly in your chest. Hold and
push harder. Release after 5 seconds.
Repeat 20 times.

Day 12

FIRST MEAL
1 small carton plain yoghurt with grated apple, juice of an orange and 3 flaked Brazil nuts
or
2 whole oranges, 1 grapefruit, segmented*

SECOND MEAL
Courgette and Tomato Gratin page 125
or
Baked or grilled salmon with a pine nut crust and mashed carrot and swede or broccoli

THIRD MEAL
Spaghetti with tomato and vegetable sauce with a mixed leaf salad of watercress, rocket, etc. and French dressing
or
2 rounds of wholemeal salad sandwiches or grilled vegetable tortilla wraps
or
Nuts and Bolts Pasta Salad page 122*
Pot plain yoghurt with walnuts

SUPPER
Winter Fruit Salad, page 138, with fromage frais*

Tip

This fortnight has been all about taking yourself in hand, and I hope you've also disciplined yourself to get plenty of sleep, stay off the alcohol and drink plenty of water. Yes, I think it's a bore not to drink. Yes, I think it's a bore to go to bed early with half a pound of cream on your shoulders and neck. But it's not permanent. This has been a rest cure, and you've taken yourself in hand. Please feel this programme is here for you to take up any time you need it. It's not meant to be a permanent way of living because that wouldn't be realistic. It is important, though, to adopt a proper pattern of grooming which fits into your daily schedule, because being on top of little beauty chores means you'll never get caught out.

Your beauty routine will open doors for you because, by feeling beautiful, you'll radiate confidence.

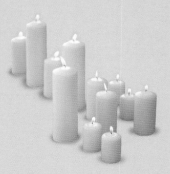

Day 13

FIRST MEAL
2 whole oranges, 1 grapefruit, segmented*,
a large latte or cappuccino
or
Fresh fruit salad with 2tbs fromage frais
(optional)

SECOND MEAL
Cottage cheese and fruit salad*
or
Lemon Paprika Chicken with Walnuts
page 111
or
2 scrambled or poached eggs, 2 rashers
bacon, mushrooms and tomatoes

THIRD MEAL
Macaroni Cheese with Tomatoes page 121
or
Vegetable curry with rice and a crisp mixed
salad*
or
Potatoes Anna with sliced stir-fried crisp
vegetables

SUPPER
Baked Banana Suzette page 136
or
Mango and grapes

Day 14

FIRST MEAL
Mixed fruit salad with 2tbs plain yoghurt
or
2 whole oranges, 1 grapefruit, segmented*

SECOND MEAL
One-Stage Mediterranean Cod page 118*
with plain steamed vegetables
or
Roast beef, lamb or chicken, vegetables,
juices from the roast
or
Cheese salad

THIRD MEAL
Cashew Nut Korma page 126
or
Two rounds wholemeal salad sandwiches*
or
Jacket potato, baked beans and salad
Portion Rice Pudding page 137

SUPPER
Mixed fruit salad with apple, grapes and pear
or
Baked Apple and Fromage Frais page 136

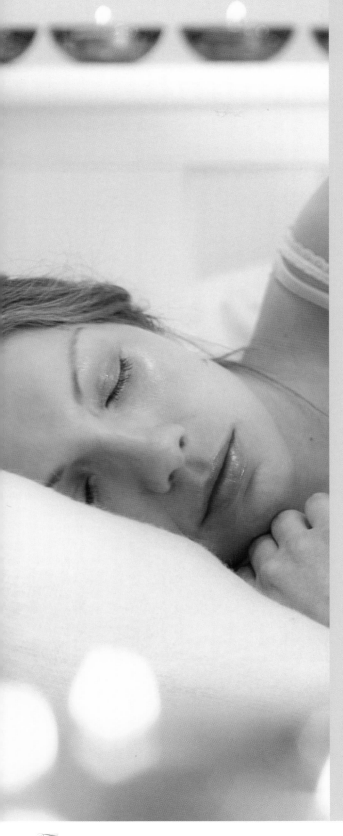

Tip

1 Is your handbag big enough?
2 Do you have tissues, cotton wool, etc., for emergencies?
3 If it is going to be hot, your feet might swell. Do you need a refreshing foot spray if you have to stand for a long time?
4 Do you have some handbag-size hand cream?
5 Have you remembered some scent? It might mask the smell of perspiration.
6 Do you need spare tights or stockings?
7 Should you carry a spare set of make-up if the day will be a long one?
8 IS YOUR HANDBAG BIG ENOUGH NOW??

The Maintenance Programme

The Maintenance Programme is for the rest of your life. We have all heard of a capsule wardrobe for busy women who need a few good pieces of clothing and standard outfits to take the hassle out of what to wear. This programme is a capsule diet and exercise routine which takes all the hard work out of deciding what to do for fitness and what to eat to stay slim.

It is incredibly important to get rid of the old you. Forget all the reasons you could not lose weight in the old days. They have gone. You have basic principles in place now. The Maintenance Programme relaxes slightly and allows you to trust your appetite. If you wish to stay on the first fortnight's programme, there is no reason not to. For general management, however, start this regime but be prepared to go back to the first programme any time you want. Some people like to do the full fortnight two weeks out of every four. Some like the food separation principles on weekdays only. Play around with it. But what I ask you not to do is eat badly at weekends, have takeaways or go on drinking or food binges. That is not part of the programme and treating your body with disrespect is not a treat for it. You've done so well so far!

Here is what to expect on the second part of your programme:

More Calories

Your first fortnight's diet allowed about 1,000 calories a day. If you want to continue losing weight or maintain your weight, you can add 200–400 calories a day as long as those calories come from nutrients. 'Empty' calories from chocolate, crisps, the odd glass of wine, etc., are a bad idea as they add nothing to your health or looks.

You add calories simply by having slightly larger portions, for example a larger chicken breast, an extra slice of toast or a handful of nuts added to a salad. I am not giving you actual calorie values in this book because it is not necessary. The programme is low-calorie anyway.

More Versatility

Have you ever been faced with your usual dinner only to find it is too much for you? You might put a plate over it and heat the rest up later. Well, this is a good idea when you want to stick to food separation but want the option of a light starch meal later. Perhaps you are going out tonight and are happy to eat the beef and vegetables but feel you've missed out on the potatoes?

The answer is simple: have them later. I often have time for nothing more than a salad at 6 p.m., especially during the summer. If I want to spend the evening gardening, it's impossible to do all that bending and digging if my stomach is full of potatoes or rice, and I can't tell you the mistakes I've made, ending up with burning acid reflux that lasts well into the early hours. So now I have the lighter, protein part of my meal an hour or so before I start the gardening and the baked potato much later. As long as there are a couple of hours between meals, it's a sensible solution.

You might wonder about eating late and whether this causes food to turn to fat. I have already touched on this, but it's worth repeating. Eating late has no effect on the body's fat storage. Actors and dancers always eat after a show, as late as midnight, then go home to bed. If you have been working hard and are empty, a good meal does no worse than replenish your stores.

Then there is the question of how late you go to bed. I am a night owl as well as a lark, and even though I might have eaten dinner at 7.30 p.m., I am usually still up at midnight. Four and a half hours is a long time between meals, so I am usually tucking into a little cereal or warm milk and fruit about 10.30 p.m.

Be sensible. If you go to bed early, you will not need supper. If you go to bed late, you will.

Easy Eating Out

Part one of the programme is hard going on your social life. I don't apologize for that, because being overweight is hard on your social life too and we all have to make sacrifices. Now you're feeling thinner and more confident, you can afford to experiment and can also probably trust yourself a little better with food. So here are some ideas for restaurant meals.

Stick to Protein Choices

As most meals centre on protein bases, even vegetarian meals, it makes sense to stick to proteins for meals out. However, this isn't compulsory! If a nice mushroom risotto or pasta dish takes your fancy, go for it! But if you are going for protein, here are your guidelines for the rest of the meal:

Starters

· no bread, breadsticks, poppadoms, canapés or appetizers
· dips such as hummus, taramasalata or olive dips with crudités are fine
· cream cheese with vegetables is fine too as it is mostly fat

Main Courses

Just leave out any potatoes, rice, pasta or bread. Eat meat, fish, cheese, eggs, tofu or Quorn. Nuts are fine with either starch or protein, plus sauces.

Try not to have two proteins in one meal, for example, kedgeree which has both fish and eggs. Look to your versatile food list for salads and vegetables that go with anything.

Puddings and Desserts

If you are still trying to lose weight, don't eat pudding! However, a little strong cheese with celery sticks will be fine. But only very small portions.

Alcohol

Do not drink alcohol if you still need to lose weight, though one glass of wine is fine. On the maintenance programme, you may have two glasses of wine per day with meals.

For every glass of alcohol, have one glass of plain water.

Here are seven days of menus which illustrate the sort of thing you can devise for yourself.

ay 1

Get back on track day
(800–1,000 calories)

First Meal FRUIT
Bowl of mixed grapefruit and orange segments
or
Smoothie made with one banana, 1tbs yoghurt, 3 slices mango and a small cup skimmed milk

Second Meal PROTEIN
2 hard-boiled eggs and salad
or
Small cold chicken breast, mayonnaise, two sliced tomatoes and a few slices cucumber

Third Meal PROTEIN
Grilled salmon with a honey and almond crust with spinach and carrots
or
Cottage cheese and fruit platter

Supper
Fresh fruit salad

Day 2

First Meal FRUIT
One banana, sliced, with mango chunks
and 2tbs yoghurt
or
Strawberry, raspberry and mango smoothie
with 2tbs yoghurt

Second Meal STARCH
Jacket potato with baked beans and salad
or
Salad sandwiches
Pot plain yoghurt

Third Meal PROTEIN
Chicken cooked in red wine with mushrooms
and onions, with broccoli and cauliflower
or
Salmon and prawn pie baked in milk with
mashed parsnip topping

Supper STARCH AND FRUIT (if hungry)
Medium-sized baked potato, 1tsp butter and a
mixed fruit salad

Day 3

First Meal PROTEIN and FRUIT
Two poached eggs with bacon, mushrooms
and tomatoes
or
Fresh fruit salad, two boiled eggs

Second Meal STARCH
Lentil soup with French stick
or
Cream cheese and grape baguette with extra
salad

Third Meal PROTEIN
Chilli, no rice, but served with grated raw
vegetables
or
Stir-fried chicken or turkey with pine nuts,
broccoli and peppers
Small pot yoghurt

Supper STARCH and FRUIT(optional)
Small bowl Special K topped with grated apple
and skimmed milk

Day 4

First Meal STARCH
2 slices toast with 2 slices cheese and
1 sliced tomato
or
40g porridge, cooked in water and a small
amount of milk with 1tsp honey

Second Meal FRUIT or neutral
Cottage cheese and mixed fruit platter
or
Large mixed salad with $^1/_2$ avocado, sliced,
1dsp broken walnuts, 1dsp sultanas or dried
cranberries, grated carrot and peas, served
on a bed of mixed salad leaves

Third Meal PROTEIN
Two lean beefburgers (preferably home-made)
with sweetcorn, peas and a colourful mixed
salad
or
Cod fillet poached in a little skimmed milk,
2tbs carrot mash, 2tbs peas
Plain yoghurt (optional)

Supper FRUIT or STARCH
Stewed blackberry and apple with crème
fraiche
and
Small portion Rice Pudding page 137

Day 5

First Meal PROTEIN or FRUIT
Herb omelette made with 4 egg whites and
2 yolks and grapefruit segments
or
Grilled kippers and grapefruit segments
or
Fresh fruit salad with 2tbs yoghurt

Second Meal PROTEIN
Plain ham salad
or
Cold salmon mayonnaise with colourful salad

Third Meal STARCH
Pasta Primavera page 120
or
$^1/_4$ vegetable quiche with salad and potatoes

Supper FRUIT
2 apples, 12 grapes

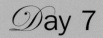

First Meal STARCH
40g porridge, cooked in water and a small amount of milk with 1tsp honey
or
2 shredded wheat with skimmed milk

Second Meal STARCH or neutral
Salad sandwich
or
Small slice tomato and cheese pizza with salad and a small baked potato
or
$^{1}/_{2}$ avocado, sliced, with pine nuts on salad with a vinaigrette dressing

Third Meal PROTEIN
Cottage pie using mince, onions, mushrooms, parsnip mash, fresh greens
or
Tarragon chicken with broccoli and spinach

Supper FRUIT
Strawberries and raspberries with fromage frais, no sugar
or
Small piece brie, 1 apple and 12 grapes

First Meal FRUIT
Unsweetened orange and grapefruit segments
or
Half a melon with grapes and a little ginger

Second Meal PROTEIN
Roast beef, chicken or lamb with three vegetables, no potatoes
or
3 rashers bacon, 2 eggs, tomato and mushrooms

Third Meal STARCH
Salad sandwiches with tomato
or
Grilled tomatoes on 2 slices wholegrain toast with mixed salad or grilled vegetables
Small slice cake

Supper FRUIT
Mango and papaya chunks with crème fraiche
or
Plain yoghurt mixed with $^{1}/_{2}$ apple grated and 1dsp almond flakes

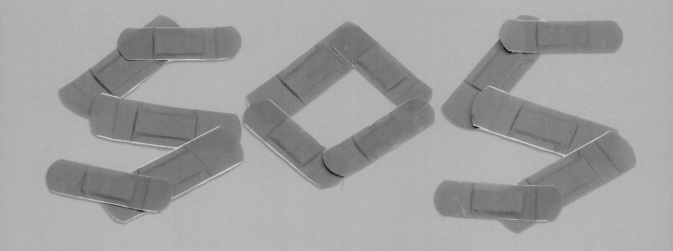

Infamous Disasters

Sometimes, despite our best efforts, a real disaster strikes. It might not seem so bad to others, but when you've spent time planning and preparing your appearance for a special event and it all goes wrong, the day can be ruined. I scoured the memories of some of my acquaintances and came up with some real cringers.

Angela, 46, sales negotiator
I was out on a first date and was desperate to hook this man! We had soup for starters and I had a poppy-seed roll. After the dessert I went to the ladies and to my horror I saw that my teeth were full of little black poppy seeds, which looked absolutely dreadful. Obviously he knew what they were and wouldn't have thought it was my teeth which were bad, but the embarrassment came from knowing he'd been looking at me laughing for a couple of hours with these black teeth. It was even worse, going back to the table with him knowing that I'd cleaned my teeth. It didn't work out.

Vicky, 22, hairdresser
I was a bridesmaid, and I had this elaborate hairdo which was all piled up on top with a twirly bit. Although we practised doing the style beforehand, we didn't know what it'd be like on the day and it was a disaster. The top bit kept falling down round my face, and I kept pushing it back up. By the end of the day – and it was twelve hours – my hair was in such a state from constantly pushing the top bit back up and trying to pin it, I looked a right mess. I wish we'd chosen something simpler!

Sylvia, 38, GP
Shoes! I always wear them in, but on one occasion I didn't and my feet were on fire by the end of a couple of hours. I was hobbling, my heels were bleeding and my tights sticking to the blood! I feel pain just talking about it.

Jacky, 31, works in a wine bar
I was at a work party, wearing a low-cut dress. I was happy and sparkling and generally enjoying myself, then I felt something scratching my chest. I put a hand up and found the wire from under my bra was curling up, and when I caught sight of myself in the mirror it just looked like a huge insect had settled there. The problem was not knowing how to deal with it, so I just held my wine glass in front of it and rushed to the loo. My biggest embarrassment was wondering how long it had been like that!

Sally, 22, hairdresser
I used to wear acrylic nails. Last Christmas my husband and I threw a big party, and at one stage I had to go and fetch another case of wine. I was opening it in the middle of all these guests, and had put my fingers under the cardboard flap to lever it up. My fingers slipped, my hand flew out and two of my nails took off across the room. At first everyone laughed, then there was silence, and those who hadn't seen it were saying, 'What's happened?' and others were saying, 'Oh, it's OK, Sally's nails have just come off!'

I still feel I can't look people in the eyes. I've given up those nails and decided to do something about my own.

What About the Future?

Anyone who spends a fortnight eating salads, vegetables, fruit and fish can hardly fail to look better than when she started. The question is, can you keep it up?

There's a difference between keeping up a sensible regime and being consumed by it. People who need to lose a lot of weight and are in the throes of a strict diet think this is going on for ever. But it's back to my analogy about buying a wreck of a house: the work is shattering for ages because you are starting from scratch, but once the place is up and running, you spend a fraction of that time maintaining it. Staying slim and shapely is a fraction of the trouble you took getting there. Remember this, once your mind is in place, your food decisions are made for you. You won't be fighting your feelings about a piece of cake if there's no contest.

This is not to say that you will never eat a slab of Christmas cake again. Of course you will. You just won't eat six slabs. The principles you have learned will stand you in good stead. Eat to your comfort level, eat when you are hungry and eat at mealtimes.

Don't get obsessed, either. Don't think that once fat, always fat. If you have lost weight, there is no reason why you even need worry about it again. Get rid of those 'fat' outfits, don't read slimming magazines (they are all about food) and trust yourself. This programme works. Stay within it and you never need worry about your shape again.

Do it for yourself, too. Let your looks enrich your life, not dominate it. Learn what feeling good feels like, learn the techniques of achieving it and then let it look after itself.

What if I go on a weekend binge?
I hope you won't do this. Bingeing is a moral question as well as a physical and mental one. But if you do slide back, keep calm. Your body won't put on weight straight away, so go back to day one of the diet plan and follow it for five to seven days. Keep off alcohol, biscuits and sweets for that period of time, but go back to the fourteen-day plan for two to three days and drink plenty of water.

Above all, don't panic or miss meals to compensate. It won't work.

If I'm going out to a restaurant for a meal, shouldn't I miss lunch that day to 'make room'?
Definitely not! If you miss meals, you'll think you can afford to eat as much as you like. Maybe you can, quite simply you have no need to eat like a horse, and it ruins the image you've been working for. Eat your normal meals, then go out and eat what you truly fancy, not what you've been saving a corner of your stomach for!

How can I look good for ever?
This is easy: follow these keys to well-being and I guarantee your life and looks will be brighter and more satisfying in every way.
1 Eat well and eat regularly.
2 Walk a mile a day.
3 Never go more than five pounds (2.2 kg) above your best weight.
4 Stand up straight and hold yourself in, all the time.
5 Relax.

A Last Word

Whatever you wear, however beautiful your jewellery, your immaculately manicured nails and elaborate hairdo, always try to smile and look as if you're happy and enjoying yourself.

If something goes wrong, if you get a drink spilled over you or the baby is sick on your shoulder, laugh it off. You might feel murderous, but people will warm to you and sympathize with you if you appear happy-go-lucky and handle a disaster with style. **Have a good time!**

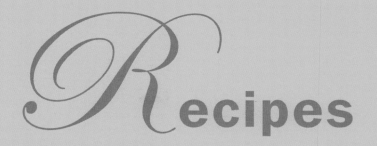

Recipes

These recipes do not all appear in the

fourteen-day programme, but you might

like to use them to vary your menus.

I have given portion sizes instead of the

numbers of people these recipes serve,

in case you prefer to make a dish

stretch to two, three or four menus!

Protein Meals

Country Chicken Casserole
4 portions

2tbs vegetable oil

2 skinless, boneless chicken breasts
 or legs

1 small onion, finely chopped

2 leeks, cut into rounds

8 small whole carrots

4tbs half-fat crème fraiche

450ml/15fl oz chicken stock

100ml/3$^{1}/_{2}$ fl oz skimmed milk

salt and freshly ground black pepper

1tbs wholegrain mustard

2tbs cream

1 Preheat the oven to 170°C/325°F/Gas
   Mark 3.
2 Heat the oil in a large frying pan, add the
   chicken pieces and cook over a high heat,
   turning, for 1 minute. Then transfer to an
   ovenproof casserole dish.
3 Add the onion to the frying pan and stir-fry for
   1–2 minutes until golden. Add the leeks and
   carrots, cook for a few minutes, then add to the
   chicken.
4 Stir in the crème fraiche. Stirring continually,
   cook over a medium heat for 1 minute, then
   gradually add the stock.
5 Add the milk, salt and pepper.
6 Pour over the chicken and cook in the oven for
   45 minutes.
7 Transfer the chicken and vegetables to a
   serving dish, reserving the sauce. Stir the
   mustard and cream into the sauce and pour
   over the chicken.

Meatballs in Tomato Sauce
2–3 portions

450g lean beef mince

4tbs pine nuts, crushed

salt and black pepper

mixed herbs

1 egg, beaten

2 x 400g/14oz tins chopped tomatoes with
   onions and garlic or onions and peppers

2 tbsp tomato purée

parsley, chopped

1 Preheat the oven to 180°C/350°F/Gas
   Mark 4.
2 Put the meat into a bowl with the pine nuts,
   salt, black pepper, herbs and egg. Mix together
   and form into small balls. Set aside.
3 Put the tomatoes and tomato purée into an
   oven-proof dish. Add the meatballs and cover
   with foil. Bake for an hour.
4 Take the foil off for the last 20 minutes of
   cooking time so the meatballs brown.
5 Sprinkle with parsley and serve with shredded
   raw vegetables or mashed parsnips or puréed
   spinach.

Lemon Paprika Chicken with Walnuts
2 portions

2 chicken breast fillets

1tsp sweet paprika

112ml/4fl oz olive oil

1 clove garlic, crushed

rind and juice of a lemon

1tsp ground turmeric

1 small cucumber, peeled and sliced into
   ribbons

100g/4oz broken walnuts

1tsp vinegar

vegetable oil, for frying

a little crème fraiche

1 Combine the chicken, paprika, olive oil, garlic,
   lemon rind and juice and turmeric in a large
   bowl. Leave for an hour or, if you can,
   overnight. Turn the chicken a couple of times.
2 Combine the cucumber ribbons with the
   walnuts and vinegar.
3 Meanwhile, remove the chicken from the
   turmeric marinade. Cook in a large sauté pan
   with a little oil, until browned all over and
   cooked through.
4 Slice the chicken, add to the cucumber and
   walnuts, add the crème fraiche and mix. Serve
   straight away with a side dish of crisp
   sweetcorn and peas.

Beef Bourguignon
4 portions

1 tsp vegetable oil

1 onion, sliced

700g (1.5lb) best stewing or braising steak, cubed

2 standard-sized glasses red wine

$1/_2$ clove garlic, crushed, optional

2 x 400g (14oz) tins of chopped tomatoes with added herbs and olives

4dsp tomato purée

6 rashers smoked back bacon, cut into lardons

500g baby mushrooms

1tbs brandy (optional)

salt and black pepper

fresh herbs

2tbsp half-fat crème fraiche

fresh parsley, chopped

1 Preheat the oven to 170°C/325°F/Gas Mark 3.
2 Heat the oil in a large pan and add the onion. Cook over a medium heat, turning constantly until the onion is transparent.
3 Add the beef, and keep stirring until it has browned on all sides.
4 Add the wine, garlic and 1 pint of water.
5 Transfer to a casserole dish, cover tightly and put in the oven for $1^1/_2$ hours.
6 Meanwhile, fry the bacon and mushrooms. Add the brandy, if using, and add to the caserole.
7 Add the tomatoes, tomato purée and season with salt, pepper and herbs. Cook for a further hour.
8 Return to the oven for a further 15 minutes. Just before serving, stir in the crème fraiche and sprinkle with parsley.

Moussaka
4 portions

1kg (2lb) minced lamb

1 onion

2tbs olive oil

1 x 400g (14oz) tin chopped tomatoes

2tbs tomato purée

salt and black pepper

3 aubergines, thinly sliced on the diagonal

tub of crème fraiche

fresh parsely, chopped

1 Preheat the oven to 190°C/375°F/Gas Mark 5.
2 In a frying pan, dry-fry the lamb until the fat runs. Remove the lamb and set aside.
3 Fry the onion in 1tbs oil until soft but not brown, add the lamb, tomatoes, tomato purée, salt and pepper and cook on a low heat for 10 minutes.
4 Dip the aubergine in the remaining oil and fry gently. Aubergine takes up oil like blotting paper so cook over a low heat until golden brown on each side. Put it on some kitchen paper to drain.
5 Layer the mince mixture, aubergines and crème fraiche in an ovenproof dish, ending with some crème fraiche on the top.
6 Put in the oven and cook for about 30–40 minutes until the top is bubbling and golden.
7 Serve with salad or green vegetables.

Chicken with Watermelon and Hazelnut Salad and Raspberry Vinaigrette
1 portion

For the raspberry vinaigrette
200g/8oz raspberries
110ml/4floz hazelnut oil
50g/2oz raspberry vinegar (a must)

1 tbs (heaped) toasted hazelnuts
1 chicken breast fillet per person
small amount of vegetable oil
$1/2$ medium-sized watermelon,
   seeds removed
100g/4oz fresh raspberries/cranberries
bunch torn lamb's lettuce

1 First, process all the vinaigrette ingredients until puréed. Pour through a sieve to get rid of the seeds.
2 To toast the hazelnuts, either put them into a hot oven or under the grill, without any oil, or into a large dry frying pan and keep shaking as they gradually turn brown. Remove from the heat and set aside – (they will keep cooking in their own oil and be extremely hot to touch, so take care).
3 Brush or spray a little oil on the chicken and grill until cooked through.
4 Cut the watermelon into chunks. Combine in a bowl with the raspberries/cranberries and lettuce.
5 Slice the chicken thinly or cut into dice, drizzle with the vinaigrette and sprinkle with the nuts. Combine gently with all the other ingredients and serve.

Salmon and Corn Chowder
4 portions

15g / $1/2$ oz butter
1 medium carrot, diced
1 small onion, diced
1 leek, chopped into rounds
225g/8oz potatoes, peeled and cubed
600ml/1 pint skimmed milk
300ml/10fl oz water
salt and freshly ground black pepper
$1 1/2$ 200g/7oz tin sweetcorn, drained
1 x 175g/6oz salmon fillet, skinned and cubed
150ml/5fl oz single cream
handful of chopped fresh parsley

1 Melt the butter in a saucepan. Add the carrot, onion and leek and stir until transparent. Add the potato and cook for a further minute.
2 Pour in the milk and water. Season well with salt and pepper and simmer for 10 minutes.
3 Add the sweetcorn and the salmon and simmer for a further 3–4 minutes.
4 Stir in the cream and parsley and serve immediately.

Chicken Roulade with Layered Vegetables
4 portions

Don't be put off by the elaborate-sounding name of this dish. Chicken Roulade is terribly simple to make and also looks very impressive. You should really blanch the watercress before using it, but I never do and it still comes out perfectly. The layered vegetables look great and add the necessary moisture.

4 skinless, boneless chicken breasts
2–3 bunches watercress (depending on size)
a little butter
salt and freshly ground black pepper
400g/14oz broccoli, boiled and mashed
400g/14oz carrot or carrot and swede, boiled
   and mashed

1 Preheat the oven to 170°C/325°F/Gas Mark 3.
2 Place the chicken breasts on a non-stick board, cover with clingfilm and beat each one with a rolling pin until flattened out to about 15cm/6in square.
3 Cut off the watercress stalks and discard. Rinse the leaves and drain thoroughly.
4 Divide the watercress between the chicken breasts. Dot with the butter and season with salt and pepper.
5 Starting at one edge, firmly fold up the chicken breast around the watercress, pressing the cress down and bringing in the sides to form a parcel. Tie firmly with string.
6 When you have parcelled up all 4 chicken breasts, lay them in an ovenproof dish and cover tightly with foil. Cook in the oven for about 40 minutes.
7 Meanwhile, layer the vegetables in a wide, shallow dish. Start with a layer of mashed broccoli, then carrots and finally swede, until you have used up all the vegetables.
8 Brush the top with a little melted butter and put in the oven once the chicken has been cooking for 15 minutes.
9 When the chicken is cooked, untie the string and slice each breast into medallions and put on a serving dish. They should look like attractive pinwheels with a green centre.
10 Serve immediately, with the vegetables, which will be ready at the same time as the chicken.

Mexican Chilli Chicken

4 portions

1$^1/_2$ tbs vegetable oil

4 skinless, boneless chicken breasts

1 clove garlic, finely chopped

1 onion, finely chopped

2 fresh chillies, finely chopped

1 green pepper, chopped

a few fresh coriander leaves, chopped

$^1/_2$ tsp ground coriander

1 x 400g/14oz tin chopped tomatoes

2 tbs wine vinegar

1 tsp Tabasco sauce

1 tsp brown sugar

1 avocado, halved, stoned and cut into
   chunks

juice of 1 lime

salt and freshly ground black pepper

1 Preheat the oven to 190°C/375°F/Gas
   Mark 5.
2 Heat 1 tbs of the oil in a large frying pan, add
   the chicken and cook on both sides until
   browned. Transfer to a shallow ovenproof dish.
3 Heat the remaining oil in the frying pan, add the
   garlic, onion, chillies and green pepper and
   cook over a low heat until just soft.
4 Add both types of coriander, the tomatoes,
   vinegar, Tabasco, sugar and season. Stir and
   simmer gently for 20 minutes until thick.
5 Pour the sauce over the chicken breasts. Bake
   in the oven, uncovered, for 25 minutes.
6 Toss the avocado chunks in the lime juice.
7 Remove the chicken from the oven and gently
   stir in the avocado.
8 Return to the oven and cook for a further 10
   minutes.

Cod in Lemon Caper Sauce

4 portions

4 skinless cod fillets

284ml/10fl oz skimmed milk

salt and freshly ground white pepper

2 tbs fresh double cream

25g/1oz butter

1 tsp grated lemon zest

2 tbs capers

2 tbs chopped fresh parsley

grated zest of 1 lime

1 Put the cod fillets in a large frying pan, add
   the milk and season with salt and pepper.
   Cover with a lid and poach gently for about
   10 minutes, until the fish is cooked through.
   Remove it from the milk and set aside,
   keeping warm.
2 Add the cream to the warm milk. Add the butter
   and lemon zest. Keep stirring as the sauce
   thickens.
3 Stir in the capers and parsley. Season to taste
   with salt and pepper.
4 Sprinkle with lime zest to decorate and serve
   with green vegetables.

Poached Cod or Salmon Parcel
1 portion

This recipe is very easy and ideal for working people who want to avoid fast takeaway food. Ready-cut vegetable batons are available from supermarkets. Use any combination of vegetables you like, but try to go for vegetables with a high water content.

2tsp vegetable oil

1 courgette, cut into batons

1 carrot, cut into batons

1 x 100g/4oz skinless cod or salmon
   fillet

7g/$^1/_4$oz butter

a few chopped fresh tarragon leaves or pinch
   dried tarragon, if using salmon

salt and freshly ground black pepper

1 Preheat the oven to 190°C/375°F/Gas
   Mark 5.
2 Brush a 30cm/12in square of greaseproof
   paper with some of the oil and place on a
   baking sheet.
3 Place the vegetable batons on the greaseproof,
   top with the fish and add the butter. If you are
   using salmon, add the tarragon.
4 Make a baggy parcel and secure loosely with
   string.
5 Cook the parcel in the oven for 10–15 minutes.

Scallop and Bacon Provençale
2 portions

2tbs sunflower oil

$^1/_2$ medium onion, finely chopped or grated

1 clove garlic, crushed (optional)

8oz fresh scallops

8oz smoked bacon, diced

5oz glass dry white wine

1 red chilli, chopped

1 x 400g/14oz tin chopped tomatoes with
   herbs

salt and freshly ground black pepper

small bunch coriander, roughly torn into
   shreds

1 Heat the oil in a large frying pan. Add the onion
   and garlic and sauté until soft.
2 Add the scallops and bacon and cook over a
   medium heat, turning occasionally, until cooked
   through. Remove and set aside.
3 Return the onions and garlic to the pan and
   add the wine, chilli, tomatoes and seasoning.
   Simmer for 5 minutes.
4 Return the scallops and bacon to the pan and
   heat through.
5 Serve, garnished with coriander, on a bed
   of grated raw vegetables or pea purée with
   a dressed green salad.

Moroccan Chicken Salad

2–3 portions

For the dressing

2tbs lemon juice

1tbs lemon zest, grated

2tbs olive oil

2 cloves garlic, crushed

2tbs mixed ground cumin, coriander, crushed cardamon pods

2tbs olive oil

2 chicken breast fillets

1 medium-sized aubergine, chopped into small cubes

2 large red, green or yellow peppers (canned or in jars), quartered

2 teacups couscous

2 teacups water

2tbs shelled pistachios, toasted

handful fresh coriander leaves

handful fresh chopped mint

1 Put the dressing ingredients into a screw-topped jar and shake. A serving is a generous 2tbs.

2 Combine the spices with 1tbs oil and rub into the chicken. Marinade for 30 minutes at least.

3 Put the remaining oil in a frying pan and heat. Cook the chicken in the hot oil until brown and cooked through. Set aside, then slice thinly.

5 In the same pan, cook the aubergine until browned – you may need to add more oil.

6 Put the couscous in a bowl, cover with 2 cups of boiling water and allow to stand until the water is absorbed. Fluff with a fork.

7 Gently toss all the ingredients in a bowl with the dressing. Serve with a green salad.

Skinny Chicken and Garden Grill

1 portion

A dish of perfectly grilled chicken on a simple salad of pan-fried aubergine, courgettes, tomato, red bell peppers and asparagus topped with Parmesan shavings.

2tbs oil

1 skinless chicken breast, flattened

2 courgettes, sliced into julienne

1 aubergine, sliced into rounds

12 asparagus spears

2 bell peppers, de-seeded and sliced

1dsp soy sauce

Parmesan shavings (optional)

1dsp sesame seeds, toasted (optional)

1 Heat 1tbs oil in a griddle pan until hot but not smoking. Add the chicken, put the lid on and turn the heat down to medium. Cook for 5 minutes on each side and test it is cooked by cutting into the breast. It should be white throughout without a hint of pink.

2 Remove the chicken from the pan and set aside, keeping it warm. Add the rest of oil to the pan, turn the heat up and add the vegetables. Stir-fry swiftly, not allowing the vegetables to stick.

3 Add 1dsp soy sauce and shake thoroughly to incorporate.

4 Meanwhile, cut the chicken into strips. Turn the vegetables out onto a hot serving dish, top with the chicken and the Parmesan shavings. Add a few sesame seeds, if you wish, to decorate.

One-Stage Mediterranean Cod
1 portion

You can use any white fish for this, for example, sea bass or sole. It is simple but incredibly tasty and ideal for the busy person – it will cook while you are taking a shower!

1 fish fillet per person
1 x 400g/14oz tin chopped tomatoes with
  herbs and garlic
1tsp capers
1 large pepper, chopped
sea salt
coriander, chopped

1 Preheat oven to 200°F/400°C/Gas Mark 6.
2 Place the fish fillets in an oven-to-table dish. Pour over the tomatoes, pepper and capers, making sure they are mixed well. Season with sea salt.
3 Bake in the oven for 20 minutes, until the fish is cooked through.
4 Serve on a bed of spinach and garnish with the coriander.

Spanish or Herb Omelette
1 portion

2 eggs
salt and freshly ground black pepper
7g/ $^1/_2$oz butter
mixed fresh herbs, chopped (for the herb
  omelette)
red and green pepper, onion, mushrooms
  (for the Spanish omelette)

1 Put the eggs in a bowl and beat lightly. Season with salt and pepper.
2 Heat the butter in a medium-sized frying pan until hot but not blackened.
3 For the herb omelette: pour the eggs into the pan and, using a fork, draw the edges of the omelette into the centre, letting the liquid run to the outside, until the omelette is just set. Add the herbs, fold and serve immediately.
4 For the Spanish omelette: heat the butter, add the chopped vegetables and stir together for a minute. Add the eggs and cook on the bottom only. Cook the top of the omelette by holding under a medium grill until set.

Starch Meals

Falafel

This is a quick and easy recipe using a food processor. For a light meal, serve with a mixed salad or yoghurt with fresh coriander and mint.

1 x 400g (14oz) tin chickpeas

1 shallot or a small onion, chopped

1 clove garlic, chopped

$\frac{1}{2}$ tsp ground cumin

pinch cayenne or chili powder

1 egg, beaten

1tbs cornflour

salt and black pepper

sunflower oil

olive oil, warmed

lemon juice

1 Put the chickpeas, shallot or onion into a food processor and purée. Transfer to a bowl.
2 Add the garlic, cumin, cayenne or chilli, egg and cornflour and mix to a paste. Season to taste.
3 With floured hands, form the mixture into small balls about 7cm (3in) across and then flatten them slightly.
4 Pour half an inch of oil into a frying pan over a high heat. When the oil is hot, but not smoking, fry the falafel until crisp on one side, then turn over and repeat on the other side.
5 Drain on kitchen paper, then serve drizzled with olive oil and lemon juice.

Pasta Primavera
1 portion

50g/2oz fresh pasta spirals or quills

1tbs olive oil

handful mixed mangetout, baby sweetcorn,
  sugar-snap peas, carrot sticks, red and
  green peppers, beansprouts

1tsp pesto sauce

2tsps crème fraiche

salt and freshly ground black pepper

1 Cook the pasta according to the packet
   instructions. Drain and keep warm.
2 Heat the oil in a deep frying pan or wok, and
   add the mixed vegetables. Toss over a high
   heat for 1 minute.
3 Add the pasta and pesto sauce. Turn for 30
   seconds.
4 Remove from the heat, add the crème fraiche,
   season to taste with salt and pepper and serve
   immediately.

Linguini in Creamy Watercress Sauce
2 portions

1tbs vegetable oil

1 medium onion, finely chopped

1 clove garlic, crushed (optional)

125ml/4fl oz dry white wine

125ml/4fl oz fish stock

1tsp cornflour

150ml/5fl oz single cream

2 bunches firmly packed watercress, trimmed

225g/8oz linguini

salt and freshly ground black pepper

1 Heat the oil in a large pan. Add the onion and
   garlic and cook over a low heat until soft.
2 Add the wine and stock and boil until reduced
   by one third, stirring continuously.
3 Blend the cornflour with a little of the cream.
   Add, with the remaining cream, to the pan and
   keep stirring until the mixture thickens.
4 Remove from the heat and add the watercress.
   You can blend the sauce in a food processor if
   you prefer it smooth.
5 Meanwhile, cook the linguini according to the
   packet instructions and add to the sauce in the
   pan. Season to taste with salt and pepper.
   Serve immediately.

Macaroni Cheese with Tomatoes

4 portions

150g/5oz macaroni

25g/1oz cornflour

600ml/1 pint skimmed milk

25g/1oz Edam or Cheddar cheese, grated

25g/1oz Parmesan cheese, freshly grated

salt and freshly ground black pepper

2 large tomatoes sliced

1 Preheat the oven to 200°C/400°F/Gas
   Mark 6.
2 Cook the macaroni according to the packet
   instructions. Drain thoroughly and put it in
   a greased, shallow, wide ovenproof dish.
3 Meanwhile, to make the sauce, blend the
   cornflour with a cup of milk until you have a
   smooth paste. Put in a saucepan and heat,
   gradually add the remaining milk, stirring
   continuously, until the mixture thickens. Then
   cook for a further 30 seconds.
4 Remove from the heat and add the Edam or
   Cheddar cheese, reserving a little. Stir until
   melted.
5 Add the Parmesan cheese and season to taste
   with salt and pepper.
6 Pour the sauce over the macaroni and stir. Top
   with the tomatoes and the remaining grated
   cheese. Cook in the oven for about 20 minutes
   until browned.

Money Bags

12 portions

100g/4oz ricotta cheese

25g/1oz Parmesan cheese, freshly grated

packet of filo pastry

melted butter

1 Preheat the oven to 200°C/400°F/Gas
   Mark 6.
2 Mix together the ricotta and Parmesan.
3 Cut each sheet of filo into 12cm/5in squares.
   Brush one square with melted butter and place
   another on top at an angle. Spoon the cheese
   filling on to the middle and gather up the
   edges, pressing them together to make a
   pouch. Brush with melted butter, place on
   a baking sheet and repeat.
4 Bake in the oven for about 5 minutes, until
   golden and crisp.

Mushroom Medley Risotto
2 portions

400g/14oz dry weight risotto rice

15g/½oz butter

1 onion, finely chopped

1 clove garlic, crushed

400g/14oz mushrooms, sliced

2tsp tomato purée

2tbs half-fat crème fraiche

salt and freshly ground black pepper

pinch of nutmeg

pinch of paprika

1 Cook the rice according to the packet instructions.
2 Melt the butter in a large frying pan. Add the onion and garlic and cook over a low heat until transparent.
3 Add the mushrooms. Keep stirring until coated with the butter.
4 Add the rice and stir in the tomato purée and crème fraiche. Add salt, pepper and nutmeg to taste and cook for a further 2–3 minutes. Sprinkle with paprika and serve immediately.

Nuts and Bolts Pasta Salad
8 portions

4oz tricolor corkscrew pasta

4oz wheel-shaped pasta

1lb fresh mixed vegetables

100g/4oz plain yoghurt

4tbs Parmesan cheese

2tbs mayonnaise

2tbs milk

1tsp garlic powder

1 Cook both pastas together in boiling water for 10 minutes. Add the vegetables and cook for 2 minutes more. Drain, rinse, and cool to room temperature.
2 Mix the yoghurt, Parmesan, mayonnaise, milk and garlic powder together in a large bowl.
3 Add the pasta and vegetables to the yoghurt mixture and toss.
4 Refrigerate for at least 2 hours.

Cannelloni Stuffed with Spinach and Almonds

*This makes enough for 4–6 portions.
I suggest you either have your own small portion, or use this for quick re-heated meals
during the week as it keeps quite well, covered, in the refrigerator for
5–7 days.*

*Despite the cream content, a small
portion of this, served with a crisp salad or
broad beans, will make a low-fat, low-calorie
dinner or light lunch.*

12–16 sheets or tubes of cannelloni

2lb fresh spinach or large packet frozen
   spinach

2tsp butter

8oz ground almonds

2tbs double cream

100g/4oz Gruyère cheese, grated

sea salt and fresh ground black pepper

8oz single cream

Parmesan cheese, grated, to taste

few flaked almonds, toasted

1 Preheat the oven to 150°F/300°C Gas Mark 2.
2 Cook the cannelloni in boiling, salted water
   until a little underdone. Drain well. If using
   ready to use pasta, ignore this step.
3 Wash the fresh spinach in several changes of
   water. Drain. Melt 1tsp butter in a large pan
   and add the spinach. Cook over a high heat,
   shaking the pan, until the spinach is half its
   bulk. This should take less than 3 minutes.
   Drain well, squeezing out any excess moisture.
   If you are using frozen spinach, ignore this
   step.
4 Put the spinach into a bowl, add the almonds
   and remaining butter, reserving a small
   amount, the double cream and the Gruyère.
   Season and mix together.
5 If using sheets of pasta, lay a 'sausage' of the
   spinach mixture on each sheet and roll it up.
   If you are using tubes, simply stuff each tube
   with 1tbs of the mixture.
6 Continue filling and rolling, tucking the ends so
   they are underneath. Grease a large shallow
   ovenproof dish with the last of the butter and
   lay the cannelloni in side by side, so they fit
   snugly.
7 Pour the single cream over the top, sprinkle
   with Parmesan and bake for 20 minutes. The
   cannelloni should be heated through and the
   cheese melted. Sprinkle with toasted flaked
   almonds and serve piping hot.

Vegetable Chilli
4 portions

225g/8oz Basmati rice

1tbs vegetable oil

1 small onion, finely chopped

1 large potato, cooked and cubed

1 red pepper, de-seeded and chopped

1 green pepper, de-seeded and chopped

handful French or runner beans, cooked and
   sliced

other vegetables (optional)

2 fresh green chillies, de-seeded and finely
   chopped

1tsp dried chillies (optional)

1 x 200g/7oz tin kidney beans, drained

1 x 400g/14oz tin chopped tomatoes

2tbs tomato purée

small dot of butter

salt and freshly ground black pepper

parsley, chopped

1 Cook the rice according to the packet
   instructions.
2 Meanwhile, heat the oil in a large frying pan,
   add the onion and potato and fry gently until
   slightly browned. Add the peppers, beans and
   any other vegetables you fancy using.
4 Stir, until heated through. Add the fresh and
   dried chillies, if using, the kidney beans,
   tomatoes and tomato purée.
5 Season and simmer gently for a further 3
   minutes, stirring occasionally.
6 Drain the cooked rice, add the butter to keep it
   shiny and the grains separated, and stir. Turn
   onto a serving dish. Top with the vegetables
   and garnish with parsley.

Cauliflower Cheese
2 portions

1 head cauliflower, washed and outer leaves
   removed

300ml/10fl oz skimmed milk

1 bay leaf

2tsp cornflour

75g/3oz strong cheese, such as Cheddar,
   Leicester, Cheshire, grated

salt and freshly ground black pepper

1 Pour boiling water into a large saucepan so it
   comes about 5cm/2in up the sides.
2 Make a cut in the shape of a cross in the base
   of the cauliflower, to allow the water to
   penetrate. Put in the pan and cover with a
   tightly fitting lid. Bring back to the boil and
   allow to simmer.
3 Reserve 2tbs of the milk and put the remainder
   with the bay leaf into a saucepan. Bring to a
   slow simmer.
4 Combine the cornflour and reserved milk in a
   cup and stir to a smooth paste. As the milk
   begins to boil, add the cornflour mixture and
   stir continuously as the mixture begins to
   thicken.
5 Remove from the heat, discard the bay leaf and
   stir in most of the grated cheese, reserving a
   handful for the topping. Season the sauce with
   salt and pepper.
6 To test the cauliflower is done, cut straight
   downwards with a sharp, long knife. It should
   feel soft but firm. Drain and place in an
   ovenproof dish.
7 Pour the sauce over the cauliflower and
   sprinkle with the reserved grated cheese. Place
   under a hot grill for a few minutes until the
   cheese begins to bubble and turn brown.
8 Serve immediately with boiled or jacket
   potatoes.

Courgette and Tomato Gratin

2 portions

25g/1oz butter

3tbs olive oil

675g/1¹/₂lb courgettes, thinly sliced

1 medium onion, chopped

1 clove garlic, chopped

450g/1lb fresh tomatoes, peeled and roughly
    chopped

salt and freshly ground black pepper

25g/1oz soft fresh breadcrumbs

1 Preheat the oven to 200°C/400°F/Gas Mark 6.
2 Melt half the butter and 1tbs of the oil in a
   large saucepan over a medium heat, add the
   courgettes, cover and cook for 5–7 minutes,
   until they are just tender when pricked with
   a knife. You may need to cook the courgettes
   in two batches, depending on the size of the
   pan.
3 Meanwhile, heat the remaining oil in a
   medium–large saucepan over a medium heat,
   add the onion, cover and cook for 5 minutes.
   Add the garlic and cook for a further minute.
4 Reduce the heat under the onion, add the
   tomatoes, cover and cook for about 15
   minutes, until they have collapsed and any
   water they give off has evaporated. Season well
   with salt and pepper.
5 Grease a shallow ovenproof dish, with a small
   amount of the butter. Stir the courgettes into
   the tomato mixture and pour into the dish.
   Level the top, sprinkle with breadcrumbs and
   dot with the remaining butter.
6 Bake, uncovered, in the oven for 25–30
   minutes, until the top is golden-brown and
   crisp. Serve immediately.

Wild Rice and Pecan salad

2 portions (one portion is 6tbs)

225g/8oz wild rice

225g/8oz butter

1 clove garlic crushed (optional)

2 cups button mushrooms

2tbs red wine

3 celery sticks, cut into matchsticks

225g/8oz pecans, halved

100g/4oz raisins

100g/4oz grated rind and juice of
    an orange

2tbs olive oil

1 Cook the rice in boiling, salted water until just
   tender.
2 Heat the butter in a large pan, add the garlic
   and mushrooms and fry gently. Add the wine
   and the rice and heat through so the wine is
   absorbed.
3 Put the celery into a serving bowl with the nuts,
   raisins, rind and juice of the orange and the oil.
   Add the rice mixture and toss gently to
   combine. Serve warm or cold as a picnic or for
   lunch.

Cashew Nut Korma

4 portions

75g/3oz creamed coconut, cut into flakes

2tbs sunflower oil

2 medium onions, chopped

2 fresh green chillies, de-seeded and thinly
   sliced

2 cloves garlic, chopped

$1/2$tsp ground cumin

$1/2$tsp ground turmeric

$1/2$tsp ground coriander

100g/4oz cashew nuts, puréed in a blender or
   finely ground in a mouli

salt and freshly ground black pepper

225g/8oz long-grain white or brown rice

$1/2$ medium cauliflower, divided into florets

100g/4oz courgettes, sliced

100g/4oz frozen peas

2–4tbs fresh coriander, chopped

1 Put the coconut into a bowl and cover with
   450ml/15fl oz boiling water. Stir, then leave to
   dissolve completely.

2 Meanwhile, heat the oil in a large saucepan
   over a medium heat, add the onions, cover and
   cook for 5–7 minutes until soft.

3 Add the chillies, garlic and spices, stir well and
   cook for a further 1–2 minutes. Remove from
   the heat and set aside.

4 Stir the cashew nuts into the bowl containing
   the coconut. Add this to the onion mixture and
   season with salt and pepper. Cover and set
   aside once more.

5 Cook the rice in boiling, salted water. When it is
   almost ready, cook the vegetables. Pour
   1cm/ $1/2$ in boiling water into a large saucepan,
   add the cauliflower, cover and half boil, half
   steam for 1 minute. Add the courgettes, cover
   and cook for 3 minutes. Drain well.

6 Stir the vegetables into the cashew-nut mixture
   along with the peas. Warm through over a low
   heat. Check the seasoning and serve, sprinkled
   with coriander, with the rice.

NOTE:
You can prepare ahead to the end of stage 4.
The coconut and cashew mixture will keep for up
to 24 hours in a covered container in the
refrigerator.

Thai-Style Stir-Fried Vegetables

4 portions

100g/4oz Thai Jasmine or Basmati rice
2tbs oil
225g/8oz beansprouts
100g/4oz baby sweetcorn
100g/4oz mangetout, trimmed
small bunch of spring onions, chopped
1 red pepper, cored, de-seeded and thinly
    sliced
100g/4oz button mushrooms, sliced, or straw
    mushrooms from a jar or tin, kept whole
1 stalk lemon grass, white part, thinly sliced
1 fresh green chilli, de-seeded and finely
    chopped
1–2 whole pods of star anise, seeds removed
    and crushed
1tbs soy sauce
finely grated zest and juice of 1 lime
2–3tbs chopped fresh coriander

1 Cook the rice according to the packet
   instructions.
2 While it is cooking, put the oil into a wok or a
   large frying pan over a high heat. When the oil
   is smoking hot, drop in all the vegetables, the
   lemon grass, chilli and star anise seeds. As the
   vegetables fry, stir them vigorously with a long-
   handled wooden spoon until they are evenly
   heated through but still crisp – about 2
   minutes.
3 Add the soy sauce, lime zest and juice and
   coriander all at once. Stir again over the heat
   while they sizzle – just a few seconds.
4 Serve the vegetables on top of the rice.

Spiced Vegetable Triangles

8 portions

1tbs olive oil
1 medium onion, finely chopped
$1/_2$tsp fresh ginger, grated
$1/_2$tsp cumin seeds
$1/_2$tsp ground coriander
100g/4oz potato, finely diced
100g/4oz carrot, finely diced
100g/4oz frozen peas
2tbs fresh coriander,chopped
salt and freshly ground black pepper
4 sheets filo pastry
melted butter for brushing

1 Preheat the oven to 200°C/400°F/Gas Mark 6.
2 Heat the oil in a large saucepan over a medium
   heat, add the onion, cover and cook for 5
   minutes until soft. Add the spices, potato and
   carrot, cover and cook for 5–10 minutes, until
   the vegetables are tender. Stir occasionally,
   and add a tablespoon or so of water if the
   mixture sticks.
3 Add the peas and stir until they are thawed.
   Add the fresh coriander, salt and pepper.
4 Cut a sheet of filo pastry lengthways into
   2 strips. Spoon the filling onto the top edge of
   one strip and make a triangle, folding the
   pastry over the filling and then turning this
   triangle down the length of the strip. Brush with
   melted butter, put on a baking sheet and
   repeat.
5 Bake the triangles in the oven for about
   15 minutes, until golden and crisp.

Salads

Spiced Lamb Salad with Mango Dressing

4 portions

2tbs ground cumin

2tbs ground coriander

1tbs ground turmeric

1tsp hot paprika

2tsp garlic salt

1lb loin of lamb

2–3 tbs vegetable oil

1 medium red and one yellow capsicum, sliced thinly.

1 onion, sliced thinly.

2 medium avocados, sliced thinly.

lettuce and coriander leaves

Mango dressing

225g (8oz) tin mango purée

juice of a lime

1 Mix the spices together in a screw-topped jar.
2 Put the lamb in a bowl with as much of the spice mix as you would like to use, for personal preference. Roll the meat in the spices until it is well covered, leave for a minimum of 30 minutes or overnight.
3 Pre-heat the oven to 200°C, 400°F, Gas Mark 6.
4 Cook the lamb in a little oil until browned all over and to the pinkness you prefer. Rest for 5 minutes then slice thinly.
5 Mix the lamb with the peppers, avocado, lettuce, onion and coriander. Mix the mango and lime juice, drizzle over the lamb and serve.

Warm Spicy Chicken Salad

2 portions

2 boneless, skinless chicken breasts

pinch of paprika

1tsp dried chillies

1tsp dried garlic granules

1tsp freshly ground black pepper

2tbs vegetable oil

salad vegetables, such as lettuce, cucumber,
    grated courgette, carrot batons, sliced
    chicory

1tbs soy sauce

1 Cut the chicken breasts into thin strips.
2 Mix the spices in a bowl. Toss the chicken
   strips in the spice mixture until well coated.
3 Heat the oil in a frying pan, add the chicken
   and stir-fry over a medium heat for about 5
   minutes, turning constantly.
4 Arrange the salad vegetables on a plate.
5 When the chicken is cooked through (check by
   cutting into a strip – it should be white, not
   pink), turn up the heat and fry until slightly
   scorched – about another 30 seconds.
6 Add the soy sauce and toss. Turn onto the
   salad and serve immediately.

Smoked Salmon and Avocado Salad

2 portions

green salad leaves, such as rocket, lamb's
    lettuce, frisée, endive

1 medium-sized ripe avocado

2 slices smoked salmon, cut into fine strips

2tbs vinaigrette dressing

1 Arrange a bed of salad leaves on 2 plates.
2 Peel and halve the avocado, removing the
   stone. Slice each half lengthways and divide
   between the 2 plates.
3 Arrange the smoked salmon strips over the
   avocado. Drizzle with dressing and serve
   immediately.

Iceberg Lettuce with Creamy Lime Dressing

4 portions

$1/_2$ iceberg lettuce, shredded

$1/_2$ cucumber, finely diced

4tbs low-calorie mayonnaise

2tbs very low-fat fromage frais

grated zest and juice of 1 lime

salt and freshly ground black pepper

1 Wash and dry the lettuce and put it in a salad
   bowl. Add the cucumber.
2 Put the mayonnaise, fromage frais, lime zest
   and juice and salt and pepper into a bowl. Mix
   together.
3 Spoon the dressing over the salad and toss
   lightly just before serving.

Bacon and Walnut Salad

4 portions

selection of mixed salad leaves

sprigs of fresh flat-leaf parsley (optional)

3tbs walnut oil

1tbs balsamic vinegar

1 clove garlic, crushed

salt and freshly ground black pepper

100g/4oz lean, rindless bacon rashers, diced

50g/2oz walnut pieces

1 Shred any large salad leaves into small pieces and mix with the parsley, if using, in a salad bowl.

2 Put the oil, vinegar, garlic and salt and pepper into a small bowl and whisk together until well blended.

3 Fry the bacon in its own fat until golden-brown. Drain well, then sprinkle over the salad. Add the walnuts. Pour the dressing over the salad and toss well.

French Frisée Salad with Garlic Croutons

4 portions

For the garlic croutons

4 garlic cloves, peeled and crushed

6tbs extra virgin olive oil

salt and freshly ground black pepper

75g/3oz white bread, crusts removed and cut into 1cm/$\frac{1}{2}$in cubes

For the Roquefort dressing

3tbs corn oil

3tbs mayonnaise

2tbs white wine vinegar

2tbs water

$\frac{1}{2}$tsp Dijon mustard

few drops Worcestershire sauce

salt and freshly ground black pepper

100g/4oz Roquefort cheese

175g/6oz frisée lettuce, torn

1 Preheat the oven to 180°C/350°F/Gas Mark 4.

2 To make the croutons, put the garlic, oil, salt and pepper and bread in a large bowl and mix well.

3 Transfer to a baking sheet and bake on the top shelf of the oven for about 15 minutes until golden. Remove and set aside.

4 To make the dressing, put all the ingredients, except the cheese, in a bowl and whisk. Mash the cheese with a fork and add it, a little at a time, to the dressing, whisking well between each addition.

5 Put the frisé in a bowl with half the croutons, pour over the dressing and toss until coated.

6 Serve immediately with the remaining croutons scattered over the top.

Salade Niçoise

4 portions

For the dressing

6tbs olive oil

2tbs white wine vinegar

1 clove garlic, peeled and crushed

1tsp Dijon mustard

3tbs flat-leaf parsley, chopped

salt and freshly ground black pepper

1 x 200g/7oz tin tuna in oil, drained and
   flaked

100g/4oz fine French beans, halved

100g/4oz baby broad beans

6 anchovy fillets, chopped

$^1/_2$ cucumber, sliced into batons

4 tomatoes, cut in wedges

20 black olives

chicory leaves

3 hard-boiled eggs, shelled and quartered

1 Put the dressing ingredients in a screw-topped
   jar and shake well to combine. Set aside.
2 Put the tuna in a mixing bowl. Blanch the
   French and broad beans in boiling, salted water
   for 3 minutes, until just tender. Drain and
   refresh under cold running water.
3 Add the beans, anchovies, cucumber and
   tomatoes to the tuna along with the olives.
   Pour over the dressing and toss gently.
4 Wash and dry the chicory and line a serving
   dish with them. Spoon the prepared salad into
   the centre. Add the eggs to the salad. Serve
   immediately.

Pasta Salad with Avocado Dressing

4 portions

100g/4oz pasta shapes

50g/2oz asparagus, trimmed,
   tips removed and stalks cut into
   2.5 cm/1in pieces

1 courgette, trimmed and sliced

1 large avocado, peeled and halved

100g/4oz very low-fat fromage frais

$^1/_2$tbs lemon juice

$^1/_2$ clove garlic, peeled and crushed

salt and freshly ground black pepper

$^1/_2$ eating apple, cored and chopped

1tbs fresh coriander, chopped

1 Cook the pasta shapes, according to the
   packet instructions, adding the asparagus
   stalks 7 minutes before the end of the cooking
   time and the courgettes and asparagus tips
   2–3 minutes before the end of the cooking
   time.
2 When the pasta and vegetables are cooked,
   drain well, and rinse under cold running water,
   then drain well again. Place in a large bowl.
3 Scoop out the flesh from one half of the
   avocado and mash it in a bowl with the fromage
   frais, lemon juice, garlic and salt and pepper.
4 Chop the remaining avocado half of the
   avocado into small pieces. Pour the avocado
   dressing over the pasta and add the chopped
   avocado and apple. Toss together until mixed,
   then sprinkle with the coriander. Serve
   immediately.

Rice and Kidney Bean Salad

4 portions

225g/8oz long-grain brown rice
salt and freshly ground black pepper
low-fat French dressing, to moisten
1 x 225g/8oz tin red kidney beans, drained
a few spring onions, trimmed and chopped
$1/_2$ cucumber, diced
2–3 celery sticks, trimmed and sliced
chopped fresh parsley, to garnish
salt and freshly ground black pepper

1 Cook the rice according to the packet instructions. Drain.
2 While the rice is still warm, add enough French dressing to moisten and stir in the kidney beans. Leave to cool.
3 Mix in the spring onions, cucumber, celery, parsley, salt and pepper and serve.

Waldorf Salad

2 portions

1 red apple, sliced
2 celery sticks, cut into small strips
20 grapes
12 walnuts
2tbs mayonnaise
lettuce

1 Place all the ingredients except the lettuce in a bowl and mix well.
2 Turn out onto a bed of lettuce and serve.

Oriental Tofu and Bean or Pine Nut Salad

4 portions

2tbs dark soy sauce
2tbs dry sherry
2tbs orange juice
2.5cm/1in fresh root ginger, peeled and finely grated
freshly ground black pepper
175g/6oz smoked, firm tofu, cut into 1cm/$^1/_2$in cubes
1tbs sesame or vegetable oil
1 clove garlic, peeled and finely chopped
100g/4oz mangetout, trimmed
4 spring onions, finely sliced
$1/_2$ head Chinese leaves, finely shredded
425g/15oz tin black-eyed beans, drained and rinsed or 4tbs pine nuts, toasted

1 Put the soy sauce, sherry, orange juice, ginger and pepper into a bowl and mix together. Leave to marinate for an hour.
2 Drain the tofu, reserving the marinade.
3 Heat the oil in a large non-stick frying pan. Add the tofu and cook, stirring, for 2 minutes. Add the garlic, mangetout and spring onions and stir-fry for a further 2 minutes. Transfer to a bowl and leave to cool.
4 Wash and dry the Chinese leaves and put into a large salad bowl.
5 Add the beans and reserved marinade to the cold tofu mixture, mix together, pile on top of the Chinese leaves and serve.

Spicy Vegetable Salad

4 portions

100g/4oz fromage frais

3tbs low-fat French dressing

$1/_4$tsp garam masala

225g/8oz new potatoes

175g/6oz French beans, trimmed

1 large cauliflower, cut into florets

175g/6oz mangetout, trimmed

1 large red pepper, de-seeded and
   quartered

chopped fresh parsley and coriander

lettuce leaves, to serve

1 To make the dressing, blend the fromage frais,
   French dressing and garam masala together in
   a bowl. Leave to stand.
2 Steam the potatoes for about 25 minutes, the
   French beans for about 15 minutes, the
   cauliflower for about 10 minutes and the
   mangetout for about 5 minutes, until they are
   all just tender.
3 Grill the pepper, skin side up, under a hot grill
   until blackened. Cover with a damp tea towel
   and leave until cool enough to handle. Peel,
   discard the skin and slice.
4 Halve the potatoes. Slice the cauliflower florets.
   Slice the mangetout into diagonal strips. Cut
   the French beans in half crossways. Combine
   with the red pepper, parsley and coriander.
5 Mix the vegetables with the dressing. Pile on to
   a platter lined with the lettuce leaves.

Spinach and Avocado in Yoghurt Dressing

4 portions

225g/8oz fresh baby spinach, washed and
   trimmed weight, finely shredded

50g/2oz radicchio washed, trimmed
   and finely shredded

400g/14oz tin flageolet beans, drained

1 ripe avocado, peeled, halved and sliced

4tbs low-fat natural yoghurt

zest of a lemon

1tsp lemon juice

fresh chives, chopped

salt and freshly ground black pepper

1 Put the spinach into a bowl, together with the
   radicchio, beans and the avocado.
2 To make the dressing, mix the yoghurt with the
   lemon zest and juice, then add the chives and
   the salt and pepper.
3 Just before serving, stir the dressing into the
   spinach and avocado until well mixed.

Bombay Potato Salad

2 portions

450g/1lb small new potatoes, scrubbed

75ml/3fl oz Greek yoghurt

pinch ground coriander

pinch ground cumin

salt and freshly ground black pepper

1 green chilli pepper, de-seeded and chopped
  (optional)

sprigs flat-leaf parsley

1 Cook the potatoes in boiling, salted water for
   15–20 minutes until tender.
2 To make the dressing, whisk together the
   yoghurt, spices, salt and pepper.
3 Drain the potatoes and immediately stir into
   the dressing. Leave to cool, then cover and
   refrigerate until 20 minutes before required.
4 Just before serving stir in the chilli, if using.
   Serve garnished with parsley.

Cauliflower, Broccoli and Pepper Salad

4 portions

100g/4oz broccoli, trimmed and cut into
  florets

100g/4oz cauliflower, cut into florets

$1/2$ small yellow pepper, de-seeded and thinly
  sliced

$1/2$ small red pepper, de-seeded and thinly
  sliced

$1/2$ clove garlic, peeled and crushed

2tbs water

3tbs lemon juice

salt and freshly ground black pepper

sesame seeds, to garnish

1 Blanch the broccoli and cauliflower in a
   saucepan of boiling water for 3 minutes, then
   drain and leave to cool. Put the broccoli,
   cauliflower and peppers in a salad bowl.
2 To make the dressing, whisk the garlic, water,
   lemon juice and salt and pepper together.
3 Pour the dressing over the salad and toss
   gently to coat. Cover and refrigerate.
4 Sprinkle with sesame seeds just before
   serving.

Cucumber and Watercress Salad

2 portions

1tbs white wine vinegar

$^1/_2$tsp caster sugar

$^1/_2$tbs olive oil

2tbs lemon juice

salt and freshly ground black pepper

$^1/_2$ cucumber, cut into matchstick-sized pieces

$^1/_2$ small bunch spring onions, trimmed and
sliced

$^1/_2$ bunch watercress

15g / $^1/_2$oz walnuts, chopped

1 To make the dressing, whisk together the
vinegar, sugar, oil and lemon juice. Season to
taste with salt and pepper. Toss the cucumber
and spring onions together in the dressing.
Cover and refrigerate until required.

2 Divide the watercress into sprigs. Rinse and
drain, then refrigerate in a polythene bag.

3 Just before serving, toss the cucumber and the
spring onions again. Sprinkle the walnuts over
them and surround with watercress sprigs.

Fresh Spinach and Baby Corn Salad

4 portions

175g/6oz baby spinach

75g/3oz fresh baby sweetcorn

2tbs olive oil

$^1/_2$ clove garlic, skinned and crushed

$^1/_2$tbs white wine vinegar

1tsp Dijon mustard

$^1/_2$tsp caster sugar

salt and freshly ground pepper

50g/2oz alfalfa sprouts

$^1/_2$ head of chicory, trimmed and shredded

1 Wash the spinach in several changes of cold
water. Remove any coarse stalks. Drain well
and pat dry on absorbent kitchen paper.

2 Halve the sweetcorn cobs lengthways. Cook in
boiling water for about 3–5 minutes until just
tender. Drain under cold running water.

3 To make the dressing, whisk together the oil,
garlic, vinegar, mustard and sugar. Season to
taste with salt and pepper.

4 Mix together the spinach, sweetcorn, alfalfa
sprouts and chicory. Toss in the dressing and
serve immediately.

Desserts

Baked Apple and Fromage Frais
1 portion

1 large baking apple

handful raisins or sultanas or
   1tsp mincemeat

fromage frais

1 Preheat the oven to 200°C/400°F/Gas Mark 6.
2 Remove the core from the apple, leaving the base.
3 Fill the centre with the dried fruit or mincemeat.
4 Put in a small ovenproof dish and cover tightly with foil.
5 Bake in the oven for 20 minutes or until soft, depending on the size of the apple.
6 Serve hot with fromage frais.

Baked Banana Suzette
2 portions

2 bananas, halved lengthways

juice of 2 oranges

1 measure Cointreau or Grand Marnier
   (optional)

2tbs low-fat fromage frais

1 Preheat the oven to 200°C/400°F/Gas Mark 6.
2 Lay the bananas in a shallow ovenproof dish. Pour over the orange juice and the liqueur.
3 Cover the dish tightly with foil. Bake in the centre of the oven for 10–15 minutes
4 Serve with the fromage frais.

Poached Pear

1 portion

1 large pear
1 glass red wine
a few cloves
1dsp caster sugar

1 Preheat the oven to 190°C/375°F/Gas Mark 5.
2 Keeping the stalk intact, peel the pear and cut
   it flat across the base.
3 Pour the wine into an ovenproof dish, place the
   pear upright in it and sprinkle the cloves into
   the wine and the sugar over the pear.
4 Cover with foil and bake for 30 minutes.
5 Alternatively, place the wine, pear and cloves in
   a deep saucepan and simmer gently for about
   10 minutes, or until soft. Remove from the pan,
   discard the cloves and pour the wine over the
   pear.
6 Serve chilled with low-fat fromage frais,
   if you like.

Rice Pudding

4 portions

*Rice pudding is equally delicious hot or cold.
The calorie content is not at all high, and
made with skimmed milk it's full of
calcium, protein and starch.*

600ml/1 pint skimmed milk
50g/2oz pudding rice
$1^{1}/_{2}$tbs sugar

1 Preheat the oven to 180°C/350°F/Gas Mark 4.
2 Put all the ingredients into a saucepan and stir
   while it comes to the boil.
3 Turn the heat down and simmer for a few
   minutes. Keep stirring to prevent the mixture
   becoming a sticky mass.
4 Pour into a lightly greased pudding basin and
   bake for 45 minutes.
5 Either serve immediately, with fresh or stewed
   fruit, or cool completely, pour into empty
   yoghurt pots and refrigerate until needed. The
   pudding can then be microwaved if necessary.
   Excellent for taking to work.

Poached Stuffed Peach

1 portion

1 ripe peach
small piece of marzipan
juice of 1 orange
$^1/_2$ glass sweet or dry sherry (optional)

1 Preheat the oven to 190°C/375°F/Gas Mark 5.
2 Cut the peach in half and remove the stone.
3 Fill the centre with marzipan and press the two halves of the peach together.
4 Put the peach in a small ovenproof dish and pour over the orange juice, with the sherry if using.
5 Cover the dish with foil. Cook in the oven for about 30 minutes. Serve hot, with crème fraiche if you like.

Winter Fruit Salad

8 portions

1 x 400g/14oz tin prunes in fruit juice
1 x 400g/14oz tin apricots in fruit juice
1 x 400g/14oz tin pear halves in fruit juice
1 x 400g/14oz tin blackberries in fruit juice

1 Combine the contents of the tins of fruit in a bowl, using only the fruit juice from the prunes.
2 You can refrigerate what you do not use for another meal. Each serving should be about 225g/8oz in weight. Serve with low-fat fromage frais if you like.